THE ANXIETY EPIDEMIC

THE ANXIETY EPIDEMIC

by

Billie Jay Sahley, Ph.D.
Behavior / Orthomolecular Therapist

Orthomolecular Research
by Katherine M. Birkner, C.R.N.A., Ph.D.

•

Edited by Alice C. Evett, M.A.

•

Pain & Stress Therapy Center Publications
San Antonio, Texas
1994

First Edition Printing, December, 1986
First Edition Editor - Alice Evett

Second Edition Printing, January, 1994

Second Printing, April, 1995

 Printed in the United States of America
Burke Publishing Company
San Antonio, Texas

Published by Pain & Stress Therapy Center Publications

Library of Congress Catalog Card Number 93-087674

ISBN 0-9625914-4-0

To my beloved mother, who is always there.

To a very special nurse
who taught me to see an eternally glowing light,
to sense hope, to find the courage to fight,
and to see the beauty of giving to mankind;
and to all RNs, members of the dedicated profession.

To those whose care and concern have filled my life
with the glory of love and strength.

And to the Lord, for always lighting my path.

Foreword

I first met Billie Sahley some years ago when we were working at adjacent San Antonio hospitals. We soon discovered many points of mutual interest, including similar attitudes toward man's physical/mental health—or lack thereof. My reading in the field of holistic medicine was avocational; I did not realize at the time that for Billie it was a part of her professional development.

Later our careers diverged. Billie set up her private practice as a therapist and established The Pain and Stress Clinic, and I became a book publisher. But we kept in touch, and it was natural, then, that we should collaborate when she was ready to publish her book on anxiety, its cause and cure.

Billie's sense of mission about her work is evident in all she does. The story of her personal experience with stress, grief, and anxiety is told in Chapter I, but there is another side to this remarkable woman which is not exposed there. Deep beneath the surface, she possesses a strength of will—a determination—which has made her face every "You can't . . ." with an "I will!" Whether this quality was developed by her childhood trauma, or whether having such strength is what helped her survive is moot. Her whole life is evidence of the positive result.

As something of a teenage tennis prodigy, Billie decided she would use this skill to get a college education. She was told, "You'll never make it. They don't give athletic scholarships to girl tennis players." But she got the scholarship and earned her B.S. degree at the University of Texas. (She won what was then the equivalent of the collegiate national title, and later, as a pro, she was good enough to reach the finals at Forest Hills.)

In 1975, I saw her open an office as Medical Marketing Consultant—the first such, I believe, in South Texas. Again she was told, "You'll never make it—and especially they'll never accept a woman. . . ." But that is how she worked her way through graduate school and earned her doctorate.

This same persistence she brings to her practice today. A patient who has gone from doctor to doctor, finding no relief from their physical and mental agony, is the person Billie reaches toward eagerly, determined that she will be able to give them the relief they have vainly sought.

There are probably other pages in her book of experience of which I am not aware, but I know she has handled hospital public relations, prepared plans for special treatment centers, developed emergency room specifications for Class I qualification, and even been a partner in a printing company. Suffice it to say that she has continually amazed me in the years of our acquaintance—and never more than the day she remarked on the phone, "Guess who got a Ph.D. yesterday?" And I hadn't even known she was working on it.

San Antonio, Texas   Alice Evett
April 2, 1986

Contents

Charts and Illustrations

Introduction

The past five years have seen a virtual chain reaction in the public's outcry for information on the enhancement of a sound mind and body. As one result, nutrition has become a true science and is coming to take its place as an integral part of health care. For years the American public lived by "you are what you eat." That has now changed to reflect the need for information about behavior, and the public is beginning to understand that "you are what you absorb."

The content of this report will focus on well-documented information and studies by leading researchers and authorities in the field of clinical nutrition, behavioral medicine, and orthomolecular psychiatry and therapy. And the point I offer you is the importance of nontoxic, natural substances to relieve stress, fear, anxiety, and phobias—most specifically, the proven effectiveness of gamma-aminobutyric acid, or GABA, for this purpose.

The forerunner in the use of natural substances to treat deficiency states and to produce a normal brain biochemistry is orthomolecular psychiatry. This therapy was first named and described in 1968 by Dr. Linus Pauling, two-time Nobel Prize laureate and director of the Linus Pauling Institute. Orthomolecular psychiatry has continued to develop and provide a successful model for treatment with specific nutrients in the diet and supplementation as required. The Academy of Orthomolecular Psychiatry is now an organization of physicians and researchers throughout the world. The Academy has published extensive research information on amino acids, minerals, vitamins, and how they affect the chemistry of the brain.

Since orthomolecular psychiatrists rely heavily on nutrition and megavitamins, they emphasize that the human body is not naturally composed of Valium, Librium, or any other of the tranquilizers so commonly prescribed today. The message is clear that **there is no such thing as a tranquilizer deficiency!** In contrast, vitamins and other nutritional factors can easily be inadequate for the body's needs, and these deficiencies can and do affect the mind and behavior.

Recently released figures show that there are some four to ten million people in the United States alone who suffer daily from dreaded anxiety attacks, fear, panic, and phobias. They swallow annually something like 982,550 pounds of barbiturates and spend an astounding $675 million for Valium.

GABA (gamma-aminobutyric acid) may possibly be the natural solution those millions of sufferers are looking for!

I
The Story of the Wounded Healer

> You can train a cold, hostile person
> until he is 93 and he will never become a
> good "therapist." Conversely, you can
> take a genuine, empathetic, warm person
> and with only a little training he may
> be a very successful "therapist."*
> *The Natural Alternative*

Originally, my search for a nontoxic medication for anxiety was a personal one, and the resolution of my own problem has left me with a sense of mission to help others find relief from their own fears, phobias, stress, and anxiety.

The episode which saw my crisis and cure occurred in my thirties, when I endured circumstances of continuing and unavoidable stress. The situation and its effects on me covered a ten-year period. It was the death of my mother which precipitated my reaction, but the story—and the reason why her prolonged illness took such drastic toll on my mind and body—actually began long before.

Psychiatry at the Crossroads, edited by John P. Brady, M.D., and H. Keith Brodie, M.D.

When I was fourteen months old, a frying pan full of hot grease fell on me and I was burned over all of my face and neck. This was in the 1930s when they didn't know much about burns as severe as mine were. In the hospital, my hands and feet were tied to the crib and I was sprayed with tannic acid. The doctors tried to prepare my mother for what they thought was inevitable. They told her that since the grease was on my eyes and my mouth and all over my head, I probably wouldn't make it because of infection, and if I did live I would have brain damage.

My mother was a deeply spiritual woman who felt that I had been sent for some special reason in her life, and she was determined that I would not die. I remember her telling me that, when she came to the hospital every day to feed me through an eye dropper and sit with me for hours.

The healing was slow, and the disfigurement was drastic until I reached the age of twelve, when plastic surgery and skin grafting could be performed. After the operation, I lay for six weeks with my head between sandbags, unable to move. I remember vividly how helpless I felt, and how I listened for sounds to tell me what was going on around me. Then I would hear my mother's footsteps and her voice, and I would know that somehow everything would be all right. I had some fourteen or fifteen hundred stitches in my neck and it took quite a while for them to heal; and it was the reassurance and optimism of my mother which pulled me through and which made me believe that having survived this I could accomplish anything I wanted.

I was living in San Antonio and my mother in Austin when she went into the hospital for exploratory abdominal surgery. I paced the halls of the hospital for nine hours that day, waiting for the doctors to emerge from the operating room and tell me whether it was a minor gall-bladder problem or the cancer we feared. Finally, the verdict: pancreatic cancer. The doctors said they thought they had gotten all of the cancer but it would be one to five years before we would know for sure.

When I was finally allowed to go in and see her, I was warned not to show any emotion which would upset her or indicate her situation. I then made the decision that she should not be told, even later, what the doctors had found, for I wanted her to enjoy whatever time she had left to live in a positive way—not dreading a disease which she had always feared.

For the next five years, I drove the eighty miles to see her three, four, and five nights a week. The stress of the situation was intensified by the recollection of the doctor's words, "You must not show any emotion." As a result, my own health began to deteriorate, and after she died I experienced a series of physical reactions to those years of daily anxiety which was devastating. Prior to this, I never had any problems with anxiety or accumulated stress; in fact, having been an athlete, I was always able to let it go ... through conditioned relaxation and exercise. Now I endured anxiety attacks and panic which ranged from moderate to severe and included the entire list of physical symptoms that occur with anxiety and phobias. Many of my symptoms resembled the deterioration I had seen in my mother's body in her last months.

When I consulted numerous physicians, I was offered an assortment of tranquilizers from Stelazine to Valium to Atarax to Inderal (all of which I refused). Nothing more ... no logic, no reasoning. They were never able to understand the post-trauma I was suffering, nor did they direct me to someone who could help me and explain what was happening to me. They could not see that I had a full-blown phobia from the extreme *anxiety*.

If I had only known then that grief felt so much like fear—the sensations were and are the same. Some of the physical problems I experienced included a fluttering in the stomach, constant restlessness, tightness in the throat, fear of choking, oversensitivity to noise, weakness of muscles, lack of energy, dry mouth, a sense of depersonalization, and a tightness in my chest so that I could not get a deep breath. I must have had five or six x-rays for this last symptom, feeling sure that something had to be wrong with my lungs. But the x-rays were always negative. Was I losing my mind?

I had test after test, all negative. The doctors were

quite willing to go on testing and offering me tranquilizers, but no one gave me any answers. I could find no
empathy, no sensitivity or compassion. The sight of hospitals brought on fear and dread, and I became almost
housebound. I did not want to drive, and if errands took
me onto the expressway northward (the route to Austin)
I would begin to shake so much I would have to pull off the
road and stop. I know now that I was "playing old tapes,"
and that my subconscious was bombarding me for all the
times I had driven to Austin under the restriction of "show
no emotion."

The answers finally came, not from any of the long list
of doctors I had gone to but from a nurse who was wise and
caring, and who had the experience and the compassion to
know what was happening to me and to make me understand it. She started me on my path to healing, started my
mind functioning. When you walk in fear, you walk alone,
unless someone else who has walked in fear realizes and
walks next to you.

Many of the patterns experienced during grief and
anxiety are related. If you can find the right help (especially when you are experiencing for the first time the slow
and tedious dying of someone close to you) ... if things are
put into perspective, then the fear does not take over. Logic
remains, and drugs—especially tranquilizers—are not
needed.

My chemoreceptors were faulty at that time, but it
was due to an overload of unresolved anxiety and grief; it
caused me to go through the helpless, hopeless state. It is
most significant that during the sixth to tenth years of this
period, from a nutritional standpoint I was totally depleted; no one really thinks of food during an acute grief
episode. And when you also have trouble swallowing, the
problem is compounded. The natural tranquilizers that
the body can normally manufacture from the nutrients it
absorbs are not there. The body is depleted due to the
malnourished state that acute anxiety brings with it, and
this condition remains as long as the anxiety does.

I could never bring myself to take any of the assortment of tranquilizers offered for anxiety, sleep, depression,

stomach pains, and headaches. I felt this would be taking more control from me and clouding my thought process, and I needed a clear head to understand what I was feeling and to resolve it so I could let it go, once and for all. The tranquilizers would have been the beginning of a long dependency.

There are amino acids which would have given relief for each of these symptoms—they have been tested in double-blind studies and proven effective. These include tryptophan, tyrosine, DL-phenylalanine (DLPA), and glutamine. Today there are products on the market which contain a combination of amino acids that relieve the effects of acute stress by keeping our brain receptor sites from becoming so depleted that we are prone to anxiety. Even children who have attention-deficit disorder or hyperactivity go through stress. Many children and adults are allergic to milk, and this is a common contributing factor to hyperactivity; yet milk and dairy products are among the best sources of the essential amino acid tryptophan.

Knowledge is *power . . . control.* If we are to be in control of our lives we must search out the needed knowledge. My own experience—the pain, the grief, and the anxiety—presented me with a challenge. I accepted this and with the help of fellow professionals and friends, I did desensitize-sensitize myself and was finally able to resume a normal life. Then I accepted a second challenge: to use my research experience to educate and inform and help others who were as lost as I had been.

II
The Nutrition
Connection

Most recent information has shown that certain drugs block or relieve anxiety and panic; this strongly suggests that the disorder has a biochemical basis. Dr. Daniel Carr, endocrinologist at Massachusetts General Hospital, states that whatever its cause, a panic attack *must* involve the brain. Dr. Carr suspects that faulty or oversensitive chemoreceptors in the brain create panic when there is no reason for it.

Dr. David Sheehan, author of *The Anxiety Disease*, reports that in most cases, his patients' problems begin in their late teens and early twenties and that although stress plays an aggravating role, biological factors may have a more important role in this disorder than stress alone. Dr. Sheehan suggests that phobias are "a real disease resulting from genetic vulnerability."

My own experience and research over the past fifteen years has demonstrated that on numerous occasions at the time of a panic attack there could be biological factors because of the physical symptoms the individual suffers. But I do not feel that biological factors are the *only* cause. Robert L. DuPont, Director of Washington's Center of Behavior Medicine, calls phobias "the malignant disorder of the 'what-ifs.'"

Many phobics can "what-if" themselves into irrational decisions and become even more helpless. Most importantly, the more control you take away from phobics, the more you feed the fear. They need control—they should make decisions, even the smallest. The Alcoholics Anonymous theory is excellent: All you have to do is get through one day at a time. Just get through today.

There is no specific single personality for an anxious person or an alcoholic. Both perceive stress differently from the average person. Any changes in eating and sleeping habits, changes in vacations and holidays, divorce, death in the family, job loss—any of these events can cause both to perceive more stress than the "normal."

In the early stages of alcoholism, the victim is often irritable, very moody, and depressed when he is not imbibing. He denies that he is drinking too much, blaming his drinking on his wife, his children, his job . . . the stress. An alcoholic sees the world around him as close, threatening, and anxiety-producing. Alcohol is the answer to all his problems, and the scary feelings disappear after a drink—the alcohol is his way of dealing with the depression and the anxiety.

In interviews with over 100 phobics whose symptoms ranged from mild or simple anxiety to full-blown phobias, the data given suggests the subconscious has become saturated by past traumatic events. These events were unresolved and continued to draw the person back into the past—to relive the event over and over but still remain helpless to change the outcome. From this stage, the chronic anxiety would develop into multiple phobias by the time the person reached his late twenties and thirties.

The key lies in the ability of an anxious person to realize, "It's over, let it go, let it rest in peace. I can't change it, the past is over, my control is in the present, not the past nor the future!" The unresolved anxiety which overloads the cerebral cortex causes the release of adrenalin which floods the brain, and the cycle of physical symptoms begins. A possibility exists that what is termed "faulty" might in fact be oversaturation from previous years of unresolved stress and anxiety.

It stands to reason if children are subjected to a parent's constant anxiety, that they too will begin to feel the same anxiety. Take, for example, the children of alcoholics—the anxiety overwhelms them. The case of "Paul" is typical.

Paul was the oldest child of an alcoholic. He cannot remember when his father was not drinking. He recalls many of the fights that his mother and father had—mostly about the drinking. He felt a confusion of feelings, including helplessness, guilt, anxiety, fear, uncertainty, and sometimes anger. He felt trapped within the family, yet he knew he wanted help.

Paul had very few close friends because he was ashamed of his father's behavior and did not want others to know his home situation; in fact, the humiliation from his father's erratic and unpredictable behavior grew into shameful feelings about himself. He was constantly trying to excel in school and everything that he did, and became an overachiever who was never happy or satisfied with any accomplishment. He drove himself, which produced more anxiety and kept him in a state of uncertainty. Paul was very intolerant and critical of others, often to the point of unreality.

His father's discipline varied between extremes of harsh severity or none at all, which left Paul in constant fear of what would happen or what mood his father would show next. He was never allowed to discuss the subject of drinking—this was taboo. When his father was sober he was very loving, friendly, and enjoyable to be with; however, after he started drinking it was as though he became a different person entirely, often becoming mean, argumentative, and abusive, mostly with words, but occasionally physically. Over the years, Paul had learned to avoid him as much as possible, hoping to prevent more anxiety and conflict. He had long since learned not to count on his father's oft-broken promises and lack of honesty.

Avoidance became a way of life. Paul found himself avoiding more and more things, always anxious and fearful that something was going to happen. He withdrew and kept mostly to himself. Over the years, as this pattern grew, he developed severe anxiety and panic attacks which manifested themselves in the form of chest pains. He made frequent trips to the emergency room but there was never anything wrong with his heart or chest. Finally he sought help for the psychosomatic chest pain and learned through therapy how his life had been conditioned by stress.

The children of alcoholics constantly bring their past into the present and feel negative about the future. Letting go is not what they have seen their role model do. Parents should learn to let their children know it is OK to show fear, it is OK to express their feelings. If they have anxiety, they should talk about it—this does not mean they're not OK. But the repressed child is growing up with the feeling, "I can't say what I feel because it means I'm weak and not OK." Wrong! They are strong and OK!

Norman Cousins, who wrote *The Anatomy of an Illness* and *The Healing Heart*, describes in detail how panic and fear almost caused him to accept open heart surgery that he did not need. Mr. Cousins follows the same path as my own: To educate and inform people is the greatest gift you can offer. When a person understands his body and the power of the mind, fear is no longer his master!

The greatest fear that all phobia sufferers have is that they won't be able to get help in time—before they lose control. *This control is dependent on the balance between the limbic system and the cortex and the GABA receptors.*

There is a great deal of evidence and research that supports the possibility that GABA has the potential to replace many of the tranquilizers prescribed for those who suffer from anxiety, panic, and fear.

In the last several years, I have on many occasions observed anxiety and phobia sufferers maintaining control when taking GABA with inositol and niacinamide . . . and *no tranquilizers*. Many of them had at one time been on tranquilizers, but as time passed they realized all they had done was traded their anxiety for pills. Soon the anxiety crept back and they had to take a stronger dose, just to make it through the day, then a stronger pill to shut them down at night, wait until morning to take the next dose to stop the shakes, the fear, the waiting for the dreaded attack. Finally someone reaches out to them and they begin to realize they want to regain control of their life. And control does not come in a prescription bottle.

Dr. Jeffrey Bland, in his book *Medical Applications of Clinical Nutrition*, makes a very important statement regarding behavior: Brain changes not only *can* cause changes in perception and thinking, they *do*. There are two main lines of evidence: 1) from diseases, which are known to distort the brain chemistry and cause the brain symptoms, and 2) from studies of hallucinogenic drugs. A large class of psychiatric patients is characterized by changes in perception and thinking.

One of the most important aspects of Dr. Bland's book is the description of clinical studies brought forth by prominent researchers which establish a new era in behavior neuropharmacology. This area of medicine now has ample evidence that nutrition can influence the production and concentration of neurotransmitters which they have equated with the action of the drugs known to influence behavior, such as tranquilizers and anti-depressants. Outlined in Dr. Bland's book are two findings that have shown how vitamins and amino acids can have a direct action on the brain receptors and clinically effect changes in mood, mind, memory, and behavior.

Dr. David Bresler, author of *Free Yourself From Pain* (and my mentor in the field of pain and stress), was one of the first to publish double-blind research information on the use of amino acids such as L-tryptophan, one of the eight essential amino acids. Dr. Bresler describes the extremely important part of our brain function that is controlled by our serotonin level; the serotonin level is governed by our tryptophan intake. When our tryptophan intake is too low, especially during anxious or stressful periods, our serotonin supply drops, resulting in depression, anxiety, pain, hyperactivity, or agitation.

Dr. Bresler states that one way to cope with this

serotonin deficiency is to supplement your diet with L-tryptophan. This will enhance the conversion of tryptophan to serotonin, thus resulting in a calm, relaxed, pain-free state of mind. The development of amino acid therapy promises to provide the body with its needs rather than merely addressing the symptoms of the patient.

By definition, an amino acid is any large group of organic compounds which are the building blocks of proteins. There are ten which are considered essential, inasmuch as they are required to be present in the diet. They are arginine, histidine, isoleucine, leucine, lysine, methionine, phenylalanine, threonine, tryptophan, and valine. These play a vital role in the brain's function. The role of phenylalanine, tryptophan, and tyrosine in depression, pain, sleep, and anxiety will become increasingly important as information about them becomes disseminated to today's educators and through the media coverage to a public which is becoming aware of the dangers of dependency on tranquilizers.

III
Causes and Symptoms
of Stress

Maria, a forty-nine-year-old housewife, felt a strange uneasiness each time she was left alone in her home. Then one day as she stood at the door watching everyone leave for work and school, the uneasiness suddenly turned into uncontrollable panic. Maria began to sweat, feel dizzy and lightheaded. She gasped for air, and her fear was over-whelming. Her hands and feet were numb. She was sure she would die before she could get to help. She managed to stagger to the phone and call her daughter to come stay with her.

That episode began a ten-year prison term for Maria. She became housebound and had to have someone with her constantly, even when she took a shower. She was seen by numerous physicians, but none was able to put the answer with the symptoms. When I first met her and lis-tened to her whole story, I had a feeling that whatever trauma occurred had been on-going for a number of years.

Finally, all the pieces came together. It had begun when she was six years old and watched her mother leave for work every day. Maria would stand at the same window until her mother was out of sight, then wait eight long and lonely hours. She was afraid to leave the house for she had been told that she could be hurt or killed if her mother was not there to take care of her. She never forgot that. When she got married, every time there was a crisis, her husband was away from home . . . and finally it all caught up with her. She never wanted to be alone again.

After Maria and I worked through all the anger and fear, she was finally able to let go, and she began to have less fear. Self-hypnosis—especially "breathing through" attacks (see Self Help section)—helped strengthen her against fear. It took a long year of weekly sessions but today she enjoys having the house to herself.

Stress is a subjective and personal affect. What is stressful to one person may not be to another. People react differently to various situations. Just because something does not cause stress in others does not mean that it might not be stressful to you.

Stress attacks can come from a variety of sources, including overwork, the death of a loved one, lack of sleep, a change of residence or of employment or basic life goals —or anything which taxes you mentally and physically. Both positive and negative stresses are taxing—even if a change is for the good, it may involve readjustments and anxieties.

Other sources of stress might be negative thinking habits, a high-strung or impulsive character, emotional drains, social pressures, conflicts, confusion, frustration, and boredom. Even certain diseases, injuries, pain, chemical or radiation exposure, and drugs can be the catalyst for stress. The warning signal for danger comes when small stresses begin to combine, multiplying their effects.

The Symptoms of Stress

Much research has been done on the physical effects of stress. Stress can slowly deteriorate the health of the body.

The first level of symptoms is very slight. They can be as mild as losing interest in doing enjoyable activities or as vague as a sagging of the corners of the eyes. Becoming short-tempered, being bored, nervous, rolling one's hands, or developing creases in the forehead—these can be evidence that the brain is dealing with more than it can effectively handle.

The second level of symptoms is more noticeable. Tiredness, anger, insomnia, loss of interest, fears, and sadness should be considered important warning signs that you are not managing your life well. Something needs to be done immediately to reverse the trend.

The third level of symptoms includes certain physical signs—headache, neck ache, back ache, high blood pressure, upset stomach, strange heartbeats, tics (facial or neck contractions), and an increased tendency to become ill. These signs can be the evidence that stress is already having a serious effect on your body.

The fourth level of stress symptoms can result in actual disease. Cancer, heart disease, skin disorders, ulcers, asthma, stroke, hepatitis, kidney failure, allergies, susceptibility to infections, pain, and mental breakdown—all of these have in some cases been related to stress.

Many times these diseases can be reversed merely by eliminating the stress. Sometimes they can be brought on by other factors but greatly aggravated by additional stress conditions. Often even the condition itself creates additional stress and therefore aggravates the condition—like the proverbial snake with his tail in his mouth.

The Physiology of Stress

Neuro-endocrine system. This system includes the pituitary and adrenal glands. Stress can so affect the brain that it tells the pituitary gland to send chemicals to the adrenal glands. The adrenal gland then produces hormones which in turn affect the entire body. These hormones in small amounts can be tolerated well by the body and are indeed necessary, but in large amounts they can be destructive. For example, over-secretions of the "fight-or-flight" hormones (adrenalin or noradrenalin secreted during fear, rage, and excitement) can lead to a heart attack or mental breakdown. Over-secretions of the "stress" hormones (cortisone, cortisol, corticosterone), caused by long-term mental or physical effort, could lead to cancer, arthritis, and susceptibility to infections.

Brain activity. If the brain cells are overworked, they can become depleted of their chemicals (neurotransmitters). Prolonged mental activity with no chance for rest or adequate sleep can prevent adequate time for these chemicals to be replenished and one ends up with a "dead battery." This depletion of chemicals can then lead to feelings of tiredness, "burn-out," and inability to enjoy life.

The autonomic system. This part of the brain controls the automatic functions of the body: digestion, heart rate, blood pressure, circulation, respiration, and posture. When the brain activity becomes abnormal, the electrical pathways divert into the automatic control areas of the brain. Thus, worry can cause ulcers and anxiety can increase blood pressure. (Do you have headaches, neck aches, or back aches? Your stress is going right to your back muscles.)

The immune system. The immune system is depressed by high levels of the adrenal hormones. However, it is also known that the immune system is affected by other factors. For example, certain "environmental stressors" such as pollens, chemicals, perfume, and even food can cause an over-stimulation of the immune system. The chemicals contained in these factors can cause profound body reactions—which we often call "allergy" or "sensitivity." This response can manifest itself with disorders such as asthma, skin rash, migraine headaches, abdominal pain and diarrhea, strange behavior, achy limbs, mouth ulcers, sinus problems, and others.

But, these same problems could result from "mental stress" as well. Certain thought processes and associations by some people can produce these or similar reactions. The challenge then is to discover which is actually the cause— an "environmental stressor" or a "mental" one. Often the stress is a combination of both, and each one aggravates the other:

➜ Anxiety ➜ Fear ➜ Panic ➜ Phobia

The key lies in control and understanding and in not

allowing situations to control you. For example, if you go to a doctor, do not pre-diagnose yourself and read your own interpretation into what he says, for then the fear will take over. By the time you get his diagnosis, you will have already developed another set of symptoms.

At the same time, the doctor has an obligation to speak carefully when he discusses your condition with you. Norman Cousin's *The Healing Heart* has the best description of the effect a doctor's words have on patients. He quotes Dr. Thomas P. Hackett, at a psychiatric convention in Montreal in 1961: "What the doctor says, how he says it, can determine [a patient's] life or death."

IV
GABA—and How It Affects Our Behavior

Human behavior involves the function of the whole nervous system. Control of behavior which is associated with emotions, the subconscious, and the feelings of punishment and pleasure is located in the base of the brain called the *limbic system*. Involved are parts of the thalamus, the cortex, and the hypothalamus.

The hypothalamus and the surrounding structures also control many internal functions of the body besides those of behavior. These "vegetative functions" include regulation of body temperature, of body water, hunger and eating habits, heart and blood pressure—just to name a few.

Experiments with laboratory animals have disclosed that the hypothalamus and the rest of the limbic system are especially concerned with the sensations of reward (pleasure) and punishment (pain). Electrical stimulation of certain areas satisfies or brings reward to the subject, while stimulation of certain regions causes punishment, pain, terror, fear, defense-escape reaction, and all the other things associated with punishment. The two systems at opposite ends of the scale greatly affect the behavior of the subject. Interestingly, the size of the punishment regions in the limbic is only one-seventh as large as the reward area.

The administration of tranquilizers such as thorazine to human subjects inhibits both the pleasure and pain centers, whereby the person is in a state of non-reality. It appears that tranquilizers work by suppressing many of the important behavioral areas of the hypothalamus and its associated areas of the brain.

Anger results from strong stimulation of the punishment centers of the brain. On the other hand, stimulation of the midline punishment regions causes many patients to feel anxiety and fear; this is usually associated with a tendency for a person to run away. Stimulation of the pleasure or reward centers yields the exact opposite emotional behavior—the patient appears calm, gentle, and subdued.

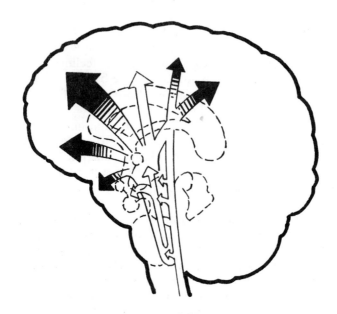

The Limbic System As It Begins To Bombard
The Cortex With Anxiety Messages

Probably the least understood part of the entire limbic system is the ring of cerebral cortex called the limbic cortex. This part functions as a cross-over zone where signals are transmitted from the rest of the cortex into the limbic system. It appears that the function of the limbic cortex is as a link to the cerebral cortex for the control of behavior.

We are all aware that stress/anxiety can lead to serious malfunctions or problems in the various organs in the body. For example, in experimental animals prolonged electrical stimulation in the punishment (pain) areas of the brain can result in severe sickness of the animal, ending in death within 24 to 48 hours. Therefore, since man is an animal, is he too vulnerable to this same type of stimulation of the central nervous system such as that produced by constant anxiety/stress?

Many psychosomatic disorders are transmitted from the brain to the skeletal muscle system. Anxiety, stress, depression, anger, or any other psychic state can greatly change the amount of nervous stimulation to the skeletal muscles throughout the body, and either increase or decrease the skeletal muscular tension. During periods of excitement, the general skeletal muscular tone as well as the sympathetic tone increases. Conversely, during sleep, muscle and sympathetic activity both generally decrease. During times of anxiety, tension, and mania, overactivity of both the muscles and the sympathetic system generally results throughout the body. This sets up a form of the fight-or-flight reaction. After a period of time, the increased watchfulness and alertness that characterizes these emotional states interferes with a person's sleep, making rest inadequate, and eventually leads to progressive bodily fatigue and mental problems.

The autonomic nerves in the body are nerves that go to the internal organs of the body; these autonomic nerves are called sympathetic or parasympathetic depending on their function. Hyperactivity of the sympathetic system occurs in many areas of the body at the same time and the effects are increased heart rate with palpitations, increased blood pressure, and increased metabolic rate. Parasympa-

The Limbic System

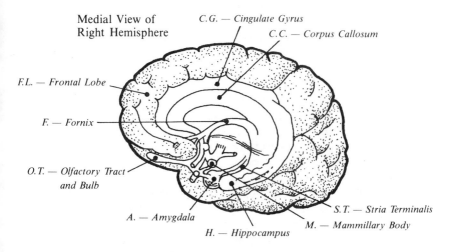

Medial View of
Right Hemisphere

C.G. — *Cingulate Gyrus*

C.C. — *Corpus Callosum*

F.L. — *Frontal Lobe*

F. — *Fornix*

O.T. — *Olfactory Tract
and Bulb*

A. — *Amygdala*

H. — *Hippocampus*

S.T. — *Stria Terminalis*

M. — *Mammillary Body*

The Limbic system includes the thalamus,
the hypothalamus, amygdala, parts of the reticular
formation in the brain stem, and the limbic
region of the cerebral cortex. Its functions deal
primarily with behavior and emotions.

thetic stimulation will generally result in more focal
responses such as increased secretion of hydrochloric acid
in the stomach leading to a peptic ulcer. Emotions control
both the sympathetic and the parasympathetic centers in
the hypothalamus, directly affecting our bodies.

Some psychosomatic effects are transmitted through
the body's master gland, the pituitary. Emotional turmoil
can usually cause an increase in the secretion of the different glands in the body; for example, stimulation of the
anterior pituitary gland causes an increase in the thyroxine
(a hormone produced by the thyroid), resulting in an
elevation of the body metabolic rate. When the metabolic
rate increases, so does the adrenalin flow which begins the
anxiety cycle.

The TV series "The Brain," which was shown on PBS
in 1985, gave a step-by-step description of what happens in

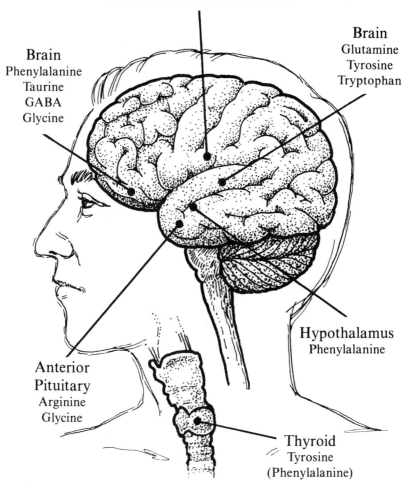

Maximum Brain Function

Brain
Glutamine
Tyrosine
Tryptophan

Brain
Phenylalanine
Taurine
GABA
Glycine

Hypothalamus
Phenylalanine

Anterior
Pituitary
Arginine
Glycine

Thyroid
Tyrosine
(Phenylalanine)

Amino Acid Direct Action
on Brain Function

GABA in the limbic system. GABA receptor
sites in the brain are like a lock and key system.
GABA fills the space preventing a bombardment of
anxiety-related messages from being sent.

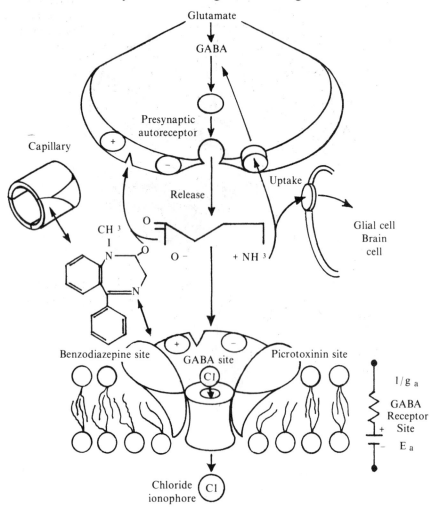

the brain to begin the cycle of an anxiety attack. Panic or anxiety attacks occur when the limbic system—the part of the brain which stores anxiety messages—begins to release numerous signals, and concurrently a physiological response begins to take place . . . the fight-or-flight syndrome and many others. To an anxious person, this is a situation of dread and fear, and threatens a potential loss of control.

The unceasing alert signals from the limbic system eventually overwhelm the cortex, and the ability of the cortex and the rest of the stress network becomes exhausted. The balance between the limbic system and the cortex goes to pieces, often leading people into erratic or irrational behavior or fear. The ability of the cortex to communicate with the limbic system—and in fact the rest of the brain—in an *orderly* manner depends critically on inhibition. GABA inhibits the cells from firing, diminishing the excitatory messages reaching the frontal cortex.

What GABA seems to do is lower the excitatory level of the cell that is about to receive the incoming information. If the stress, panic, fear, etc., is prolonged, GABA's ability to block the messages is decreased, and finally the process by which the signals are rated for priority breaks down and the frontal cortex is literally bombarded with anxiety messages. There follows a full-blown panic attack.

With the limbic system firing broadside fight-or-flight signals at the frontal cortex, the subject's ability to reason is diminished. The effects now can include fear of dying, pounding heart, sweating, trembling, tightness, weakness, loss of control, disorientation—the list is endless. Research has shown that GABA taken with inositol and niacinamide can actually mimic the tranquilizing effect of Valium and Librium but without the heavy sedated effect of these drugs. This information was first released for publication in 1982 in *Life Extension* by Sandy Shaw and Durk Pearson. Since that time, numerous studies have been published showing the successful use of GABA with anxiety-prone individuals and phobics.

Research reports have shown that a person who constantly experiences 'what-if'-type anxiety, or what is termed 'anticipatory fear,' has empty GABA receptors in the brain. This means that the brain can be bombarded with random firings of excitatory messages. It is the receptor site in the brain that prevents the reception of all the random firings so that the brain does not become overwhelmed. In *Lancet*, August 14, 1982, a research report about tranquilizers and GABA transmission clearly stated that GABA is a major inhibitory transmitter in the mammalian central nervous system and that the agents that raise the brain's GABA concentration possess a sedative anti-convulsant property.

After publication of information on GABA in *Life Extension*, the public quickly became aware of the potentiality of GABA as an anti-anxiety formula. Twinlabs, Inc., one of the largest vitamin manufacturers in the world, began producing GABA for sale and distribution. Survey of the medical journals shows over 300 articles (case studies, clinical reports, etc.) on GABA by orthomolecular psychiatrists and researchers.

GABA, and the neurons that utilize it as an inhibitory transmitter, is found throughout the central nervous system. In view of our growing knowledge regarding the regulation of the physiology of the central nervous system, GABA is assuming an ever-enlarging role as a major influence on drugs, in many cases replacing them, e.g., DLPA and tyrosine. Preliminary pharmacological and clinical data have already demonstrated the usefulness of GABA in exploring human disease.

Dr. K. J. Bergman at Mt. Sinai School of Medicine published an extensive review in *Clinical Neuropharmacol* (1985) titled "Progabide: A New GABA Mimetric Electric Agent in Clinical Use." Dr. Bergman sums up the research and results of the clinical chemistry, the role of GABA, and the influences in the central nervous system. The most valid research published on GABA relates to anxiety.

Scott M. Fishman and David Sheehan, M.D., published a report in *Psychology Today* (April 1985) stating that as many as ten million people in the U.S. alone suffer from such anxiety or panic attacks with little or no warning and for no apparent reason. Anxiety/panic attacks can occur at any time, when a person is walking, working, resting, shopping, driving. There is virtually no warning prior to the start of the symptoms.

Attacks which repeatedly occur in a particular situation begin to form a pattern, and a person will come to avoid that place or situation because they think the cause is centered around that point. This is called "situational anxiety." If the person continues to withdraw, gradually the avoidance develops into a phobia, and as he begins to avoid more and more places because of the fear of attacks, he becomes homebound—the only place he feels safe.

The variety of symptoms which characterize anxiety and panic attacks is extremely difficult for a physician to diagnose. Fear (the strongest emotion in our bodies) and anxiety and panic can all control our action and they can disguise themselves in physical symptoms ranging from rapid heartbeat or heart attack to every known medical specialty. Phobia sufferers will usually run the gamut before they finally figure out their problem, or until someone steers them in the right direction, or they are put in touch with educational information or resources pertaining to GABA.

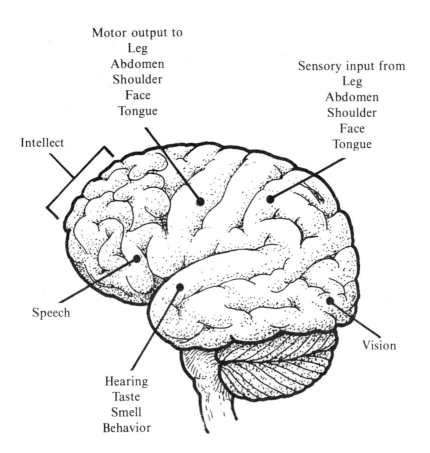

Motor output to
Leg
Abdomen
Shoulder
Face
Tongue

Sensory input from
Leg
Abdomen
Shoulder
Face
Tongue

Intellect

Speech

Vision

Hearing
Taste
Smell
Behavior

Each area of the brain controls particular activities.
Generally, the outer and forward areas serve
more advanced functions: the inner structures
determine basic metabolic processes. Each side of the
brain receives the sensory impressions and
activates the muscles of the opposite side of the body.

Thalamus

Takes in conscious sensory
stimuli (excluding taste) and
relays them to specialized
sensory areas on the cerebral cortex.

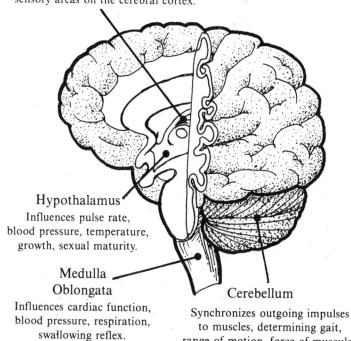

Hypothalamus
Influences pulse rate,
blood pressure, temperature,
growth, sexual maturity.

Medulla
Oblongata
Influences cardiac function,
blood pressure, respiration,
swallowing reflex.

Cerebellum
Synchronizes outgoing impulses
to muscles, determining gait,
range of motion, force of muscular
contraction, and coordination.

New studies indicate a difference in blood flow
between the right and left sides of a specific brain area
may cause panic attacks. Panic attacks seem to
occur in the region of the brain believed to control
emotions. The difference in blood flow between
hemispheres is probably connected with
differences in metabolic rate. Panic disorders could
result when a hormone or neurotransmitter
that normally regulates anxiety is missing
or deficient.

Source Daniel Carr, M.D. Massachusetts General Hospital.

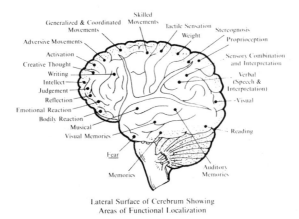

Lateral Surface of Cerebrum Showing
Areas of Functional Localization

The Human Brain

Most recently published in the April, 1985 issue of *Psychology Today*, psychiatrist, Ferris Pitts at Southern California School of Medicine found a build-up or outpouring of lactate in the bloodstream could cause anxiety attacks, or that an individual's behavior pattern would become disorganized.

Panic or anxiety attacks occur when the limbic system, an integral part of the brain which stores anxiety messages, begins to release numerous signals and a physiological response begins to take place— the "Fight or Flight Syndrome." To an anxious person, this is a situation of dread, fear, and a potential loss of control. As this occurs, so does the number of signals.

The human body functions as an interdependent, coordinated unit. Its activities, actions and reactions are directed by the brain through the vast and complex network of the nervous system. The brain itself is the most complex and the largest mass of nervous tissue present in the body, and directs the complex activities of the body. Through the five senses—touch, sight, smell, taste, and hearing—the brain keeps each of us in touch with conditions and events in the world around us.

The human body performs two basic types of movement or action: voluntary and involuntary (reflex). In a voluntary action

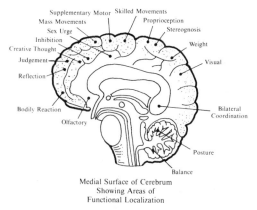

Medial Surface of Cerebrum
Showing Areas of
Functional Localization

the brain calls upon the muscles or organs of the body to perform a task. In a reflex or involuntary action the senses communicate a condition or situation to the brain, and the brain responds by calling upon motor nerves to react or respond to the stimulus. In reflex actions the brain is often bypassed, and the sensory nerve may call upon the motor nerve directly, thru the spinal cord, or in direct contact with the motor nerve. Reflex actions do not require thought or "brain-work" for the reaction to occur.

Most of the nerves that activate the muscles of the body stem from the spinal cord. The cord runs up the spine and enters the skull cavity through an opening at the base of the cranium. It then expands and fills the skull cavity to form the "brain." The organ we generally term as the "brain" consists of five connected but distinct parts—the cerebrum, the mid-brain, the cerebellum, the pons, and the medulla oblongata.

The weight of the brain of the adult male is approximately 48.6 ounces, and the adult female about 44 ounces. In the human embryo the brain first consists of three sections, the forebrain, the midbrain, and the hindbrain. As the embryo develops, the brain forms and develops its other parts. Growth continues very rapidly up to the fifth year, then continues more slowly until about the twentieth year, and then in advanced age gradually loses weight.

The largest section of the brain is the cerebrum, which is divided into two sections, the left and right cerebral hemispheres. The ability of man to remember and utilize past experience, to cope with current situations—to think and to reason—differentiate him from and raise him above the animal.

MINERAL NAME	WHERE FOUND IN BODY	USED BY BODY FOR	FOOD SOURCES	DEFICIENCY SYMPTOMS	COMMENTS

Calcium	bones) 99%
	teeth)
	fluids
	tissues
		activates enzymes
		intercellular osmosis
		blood clotting
		heart & muscle
		  contraction
		calm nerves
			bone meal
			milk
			cheese
			green vegetables
				osteoporosis
				osteomalacia
				slow nerve impulse
				  & response
				muscular cramps &
				  convulsions
				heart palpitations
				slow pulse
					Must be in balance with phosphorus at a ratio of 2:1; this balance is also enhanced by Vitamin D

Phosphorus	bones - 66%
	all body cells
		protein, carbohydrate
		  & fat synthesis
		muscular contractions
		secretion of hormones
		nerve impulses
		kidney function
		neutralizes blood acidity
			bone meal
			egg shells
				loss of appetite
				  and weight
				nervousness
				mental sluggishness
				fatigue
					Calcium-phosphorus balance is upset by ingestion of sugar

Iron	red blood cells	oxygen absorption in blood respiratory action	egg yolks green vegetables raisins molasses liver	anemia poor memory sore mouth & lips	
Sulphur		glossy hair smooth skin secretion of bile healthy fingernails	fish eggs cabbage beef Brussel sprouts		

Mineral		Function	Sources	Deficiency	Notes
Iodine	Thyroid = 2/3 Blood & tissues = 1/3	fat utilization	kelp salmon onions	goiter obesity sluggish metabolism lowered mentality dry, brittle hair rapid pulse & palpitations tremors & nervousness restlessness irritability	
Sodium		maintains acid-base balance normal fluid balance nerve reactions muscular contractions blood & lymph health keeps other minerals in solution carbohydrate metabolism use of amino acids digestive secretions	sea food poultry celery squash beets carrots chard	gas weight loss muscle shrinkage susceptibility to heat exhaustion	Works with potassium for proper acid-alkaline balance. Mostly found outside cells.
Potassium		normalizes heart beat healthy muscles oxygen absorption by brain waste disposal by kidneys water balance	citrus fruits figs bananas mint peppers molasses	edema constipation nervousness insomnia slow & irregular heart enlarged kidneys	Works with sodium. Mostly found inside cells. Too much salt destroys balance.

MINERAL NAME	WHERE FOUND IN BODY	USED BY BODY FOR	FOOD SOURCES	DEFICIENCY SYMPTOMS	COMMENTS
Magnesium	bones = 10% tissues muscles blood	relaxed nerves body cooling co-enzyme in protein building carbohydrate metabolism	beet greens sunflower seeds cucumbers cauliflower figs lemons grapefruit nuts	nervousness sensitivity to noise	
Copper		converts iron into hemoglobin utilization of vitamins	almonds beans peas whole wheat prunes liver egg yolks shrimp	lameness anemia bone fractures sores on skin weakness respiratory impairment schizophrenia	
Chlorine		stimulates liver production of hydro-chloric acid flexible joints & tendons distribution of hormones	kelp dulse leafy green rye	hair & tooth loss poor digestion weak muscular con-traction	
Fluorine	all tissues		most sources listed above		Excess in diet may cause weak bones & mottled teeth.

Zinc	semen insulin pancreas	storage of glycogen tissue respiration sparks vitamin action male hormone intestinal absorption of foods carbohydrate utilization	liver meat foods listed above	retarded growth retarded sex development rough skin poor appetite mental lethargy impaired sense of taste poor wound healing susceptibility to infections
Manganese	liver	assimilation of Vitamin B strong bones enzyme action strong nerves promotes lactation	green leaves peas beets egg yolks grains sunflower seeds	laziness impotence sterility

Anatomy of the Brain

The Meninges are the three coverings which lie between the skull and the brain.

1) The DURA MATER is the tough, fibrous membrane, rough on the outer surface and smooth on the inner surface, furnishing protection to the brain. It contains many arteries, veins, and sensory nerves, and projects into the cranial cavity to divide it into partitions. The falx cerebri separates the cerebral hemispheres, the falx cerebelli partially separates the cerebellar hemispheres, and the tentorium cerebelli separates the cerebrum and the cerebellum.

2) The middle layer, the ARACHNOID MEMBRANE consists of bundles of blended fibrous and elastic tissue. There is a space between it and

3) the PIA MATER filled with the cerebrospinal fluid, called the subarachnoid cavity. The pia mater is the inner layer which dips into the convolutions of the brain. It consists of small arteries and veins with connective tissue which furnish the blood supply of the brain.

The Lateral Ventricles are spaces within the cerebral hemispheres of the forebrain, filled with cerebrospinal fluid. As the brain develops from the embryo, the walls of the forebrain thicken and form the thalami and the cavity or space is reduced in size to a slit known as the third ventricle.

The Midbrain, as the nervous system develops, has a thickening of its walls, which develop into two cylindrical bodies, the cerebral peduncles, and its central cavity also is reduced to a narrow canal called the cerebral aqueduct. On the rear or dorsal wall, two pair of rounded protuberances develop, the corpa quadrigemina, anterior and posterior.

The Hindbrain includes the pons in the frontal section above the medulla or bulb and in front of the cerebellum. The pons is made up of a connecting bridge of fibers which connect the halves of the cerebellum, joining the midbrain with the medulla below it. The medulla lies between the pons and the spinal cord and contains such vital centers as the respiratory, vasomotor and cardiac centers. In the hindbrain is a large cavity, the fourth ventricle, which connects with the cerebral aqueduct above, and with the central canal of the spinal cord below.

The Spinal Cord contains nerve cells along its entire length, and has bundles of long nerve processes, or nerve trunks, extending to different parts of the medulla, pons, midbrain and cerebrum.

The Cerebellum, largest part of the hindbrain, lies in the posterior cranial fossa. It is covered by the layer of dura mater called the tentorium, which also serves to separate it from the posterior section of the cerebrum. It is composed of two hemispheres and a middle section or lobe between them, called the vermis. The bands of fibers, peduncles, connect the brain stem to the cerebellum. The superior cerebellar peduncle connects the midbrain, the middle cerebellar peduncle with the pons, and inferior cerebellar peduncle with the medulla. The cerebellum functions as a reflex center for coordination and degree of voluntary movements. Damage to the cerebellum affects coordination, but as reeducation of the motor areas occurs, it is clear that voluntary movements are coordinated in the cerebellum, but do not originate there.

The Cerebrum is the largest part of the brain and is the center of intelligence, sensation, the emotions, and volition memory. It is divided into two hemispheres, right and left, by the longitudinal fissure. Each hemisphere is made up of an outer coating, the cerebral cortex (gray matter) covering an inner mass of white matter. Within each hemisphere is a space (ventricle) connecting with the third ventricle thru an opening called the Munro foramen. These spaces within the hemispheres are called the lateral ventricles. Each hemisphere has five lobes: frontal, parietal, temporal, occipital, and insula. Injury or stimulus to any part of the cerebrum has its effect in the movement or action of the opposite side of the body.

The Cortical Areas control particular motor, sensory and association responses. 1) The Post Central Area is concerned with sensory activity, touch, and muscle. In the occipital lobe we find the visual center, in the superior temporal convolution the auditory center, in the hippocampal area the taste and smell centers. 2) The Frontal Area has to do with association of ideas, conduct and behavior, and intellectual concentration. 3) The Precentral areas have to do with voluntary movement and exercise volitional control over the skeletal muscles. In the front of this area is a psychomotor area which is concerned with carrying out skilled acts.

The Cerebral Nuclei, or Basal Ganglia, are gray masses deep in the white matter of the cerebral hemispheres. The most important are the thalamus and the corpus striatum. The thalamus is an oval shaped body, in two parts which are separated by the third ventricle area, and connected with a stretch of gray matter termed the massa intermedia. It appears that the thalamus functions as a center for crude and uncritical sensation and response, and in most animals it is the highest sensory response area, making their sensations primitive and imperfect. In man the thalamus passes fresh relays of nerve fibre to the cerebral cortex, where finer interpretations and reactions enter conscious sensation. The corpus striatum has not yet been clearly defined as to function, but seems to exert an effect on and steadies voluntary movement without initiating such movement.

The Hypothalamus is found below the thalamus and forms the bottom and a portion of one wall of the third ventricle. It holds the temperature control centers of the body, one center for controlling heat loss functions thru sweating and panting is found in the anterior (frontal) section, and the other section for preventing heat loss and increasing heat production is found in the posterior (rear) section. It also plays a part in the metabolic process through a connection with the posterior lobe of the pituitary gland.

V

The Nature of
Fear and Phobias

Spontaneous panic attacks—those that happen for no apparent reason—have multiple symptoms. When this happens to a person, he is so overwhelmed by fear that he begins to hyperventilate and lose all reality and reason—his only thought is to get help.

John was driving on the expressway the first time he had an attack. He headed for the nearest hospital emergency room. As soon as a doctor appeared, John began to describe his feelings:

> My heart is racing . . . it's banging. I can feel it in my throat . . . I know I'm missing heartbeats . . . I have a constant sharp pain under my heart. My hands are sweaty and limp. I feel like I have pins and needles sticking in my hands (or head). I'm choking . . . I can't take a deep breath . . . my chest is so tight. I feel like I have ants crawling all over me sometimes and I want to get up and run, but I don't know where. There is a tight band, almost like steel, around my head, and this ringing in my ears, and my vision blurs. I have diarrhea. I can't sleep . . . I wake up in the middle of the night for

no reason . . . I don't know what's wrong . . . Am I
going to die? I'm depressed . . . I feel dreadful. I
have this terrible fear that I'm going to lose control. My mouth is dry . . . Am I having a heart
attack? The muscles in the back of my neck are
like boards.

Typically, the emergency room physician checked
John over completely. When he was sure all was in order
physically, he gave John a tranquilizer and told him he was
under too much stress—and sent him home. There was no
way the emergency room doctor was going to be able to
convince John that his problem was emotional. This was
his first encounter with the chemical straitjacket; many
more would follow before he found a therapist who detox-
ified him (took him off tranquilizers) and began to teach
him the nature of panic. He learned that spontaneous
panic comes from nowhere, and can last for varied periods
of time, and may strike anytime. With a combination of
natural substances and empathetic discussions, the therapist helped him to understand and overcome his panic.

Today there is much information on anxiety available
to physicians—not distributed by drug salesmen and not
requiring a prescription, but effective. The Academy of
Orthomolecular Psychiatrists documented thousands of
cases in medical journals discussing mental and physical
reactions when the brain is deprived of essential nutrients.
This subject is dealt with in detail in *A Physician's Handbook of Orthomolecular Medicine*, published in 1979.

Most phobics will start with a spontaneous panic
attack, the severity of which can be dependent on nutrient
deficiency in the brain. If there has been alcohol consumption on a regular basis, the deficiencies will be more pro-
nounced.

Agoraphobics, those who have a multitude of fears
and avoid everything possible, will focus on their health,
and fear of loss of control while driving—afraid of not
being able to get help in time should something happen.
Agoraphobics have a lot of free-floating anxiety; they are
not sure what they are afraid of, but it seems as though

they are afraid of everything.

Fear is the essence of anxiety! Simple or mixed phobias will cause anxiety and some panic, but they focus mainly on specific objects, e.g., expressways, driving, water, heights, flying, bridges, dentists . . . again, whatever they feel will take control away from them.

A fear is termed irrational when the sufferer has had ample time to learn that a situation is not as dangerous as he had initially thought but he still persists in avoidance. The only way to conquer fear is to challenge it. Do something about it, minimize the danger, and the anxiety goes away, even though there is still some danger there. That is the major reason fear persists. The experience of anxiety is the experience of inaction in the face of dangerous situations.

"Lisa" was a typical phobic—firmly convinced that she had some incurable disease. But when she was examined from head to toe and told nothing was wrong she reacted vigorously because she was sure the physician had missed something. So she went to another physician, had another test . . . still negative. Soon she was on a steady diet of tranquilizers, dependent on them to control the fear. She was defining herself as someone too afraid to function alone. Only by not giving in to fear could she define herself as someone who was ready and able to benefit from an experience.

Tranquilizers encourage a passive approach to existence. If you are afraid of flying and take pills, you'll never learn to just relax and let time pass and enjoy the flight. Flying represents the loss-of-control factor—that's what sets off the fear. Then why not be afraid on a bus or train?

Anticipatory fear and anxiety is related to a situation of being suspended in time without knowing your future. Example: waiting for results of a test, you imagine you have failed, been fired—all the bad things you can think of. This can set up a fear cycle about tests. If worrying about the future would change it, then we should all take one hour a day to sit and worry.

There is one kind of stress which is "normal"—the result of a death in the family, divorce, job loss, etc. This is called *exogenous* anxiety and is a reaction to unavoidable, outside situations.

Endogenous anxiety, on the other hand, is the kind that comes with fear and panic—the panic attacks which can come at anytime. Endogenous anxiety is thought to be biological, but there are many variables to this theory. True, the attacks are internal in origin, but if the GABA receptors are full, then the limbic system cannot bombard the cerebral cortex with anxiety because the GABA sets up a screen and slows down the excitatory messages.

Generally, a patient who is having panic attacks is likely to have underlying phobias. A person can develop a fear of a particular place or situation, and this is generally the circumstance that brings on the attack. Phobias can be very crippling, and the victim emphasizes the unpredictability of when the attack will occur, so he anticipates and suffers a lot of anticipatory anxiety. "What is going to happen if . . .?" "And what if that . . .?" And he will actually talk himself into attacks. Until I understood this in my own case, I subconsciously programmed myself daily, even to exact times of the day the attack would occur.

This is why one might say that panic and fear and phobia attacks are psychosomatic in origin. Fear is the most powerful emotion of all. Fear overrides anything else within the body. And what organ is stressed and is called upon when a person has fear? The adrenal glands. Putting your body under a tremendous amount of fear-stress causes the release of a lot of epinephrine and norepinephrine. The body becomes depleted of all neurotransmitters, and you are nutritionally and emotionally a wreck.

Many patients I have treated have either been to one or two emergency rooms or have seen four or five doctors. They are usually on a whole regimen of medications which they hope will control some of their symptoms and relieve them of some of their anxiety. They may be taking anything from Tofranil to Nardil and Xanax. Some are even placed on Inderal, Ativan, or Valium. All kinds of tranquilizers. But to date, there has been no specific drug that relieves fear as effectively as a therapist who understands what it is you are afraid of—helping you to confront it and let it go. Because no specific drug has become traditional for anxiety and phobias, many psychiatrists prescribe whatever has been given to them by the drug salesman. Traditional medicine believes that drug therapy is far superior to talk therapy. But no study has ever shown that drugs have the same effect as an empathetic voice that understands because he or she too has been there and understands the face of fear.

One of the most unusual cases I have treated was a thirty-year-old male, "Woody," who was referred to me by his psychiatrist. His major complaint was fear of food—*any* food—unless he prepared it himself. The initial in-depth interview showed that he had multiple phobias and was agoraphobic. He was also extremely thin and suffering from malnutrition.

The food phobia started after a case of food poisoning from eating tainted chicken. Woody was alone at the time and he had the "blind staggers" and felt he was dying. This precipitated an intense fear of having a recurrence.

I went back with him to the age of eight years and found that his mother had been a very strong factor in his life. She constantly used the negative images that projected fear. No matter what he did, her outlook was the negative side emphasizing hurt, pain, and possible death. Woody's phobias stemmed from the constant bombardment of these negative images. His fixation, or phobic fear, equalled out to a loss of control, but specifically the "helpless-hopeless" feeling. The basic focus of his fear was death.

In discussing death with me, he stated that he had had an intense fear of dying since early childhood. A string of accidents had reinforced the fear.

At fifteen, after a near-fatal car accident he insisted that despite his serious injuries he must go home so that his mother could see him—he feared that a phone call from the emergency room would give her a heart attack.

Trapped in an outside elevator, he became so

panicky that he pried the doors open and jumped out. Fortunately he was only four floors up, for he would have jumped if it had been twenty.

Another teenage trauma involved crawling over a large area of dead bats while repairing his house. Three weeks later, he was thoroughly convinced that he had rabies and was dying, despite every reassurance the doctors could give him.

Working in an oil refinery brought several major traumas; e.g., he was sprayed in the eyes with a chemical and told he would be permanently blind; he was blown off a stand by hot steam. And then came the food poisoning episode.

Woody's phobias had multiplied and diversified as he matured. He developed fear of height, fear of blindness, fear of loss of control, fear that he couldn't get to help in time. The episode which had indirectly brought him to me was waking up in the middle of the night in a state of panic —rapid heartbeat, fear of a heart attack, sweaty palms, gasping, hyperventilating, and afraid of passing out.

Basically, Woody had been traumatized by all these events and never allowed to deal with his fears. The process of treatment involved no tranquilizers, no drugs. He was provided information on food supplements to repair his physical depletion, and taught conditioned relaxation exercises, the "nothing is going to happen" routine, and how to "breathe through" an anxiety attack. His wife was told the cause and character of his phobias, and she learned how to help him. In two months he was not only eating food cooked by his family but going to restaurants regularly with no problem. The panic attacks were gone and he was physically rejuvenated.

Many patients on first interview are very depressed and have a dejected mien. They actually have a deficiency in their serotonin level. On the other hand, a severe deficiency in children results in hyperactivity and mania and behavior disorders; they can be irritable and overexcited. It all depends on a person's individual identity.

Our neurotransmitters are vitally important. If we do not get the precursors in our diet (namely, the catecholamines: tyrosine, acetylcholine, choline, serotonin, and tryptophan), the neurons cannot manufacture the neurotransmitters. They all have to be made from the precursors. The neurotransmitters control our behavior by reacting on specific receptors in the brain, such as GABA, which would fill the receptor sites and keep the limbic system from overwhelming the cortex with anxiety messages. Norepinephrine is a particular hormone needed to control problems of anxiety and depression. The presence of the amino acid tyrosine creates biological reactions which stimulate certain glands in the body to release norepinephrine and eliminate depression.

According to Dr. Alan Gelenberg and Richard J. Wurtman of the Department of Psychiatry at Harvard Medical School, the basic cause of depression may be a deficiency of norepinephrine transmission at specific locations in the brain. A study in the effective use of tyrosine for the treatment of depression was published in the May 1980 issue of the *American Journal of Psychiatry*. The Huxley Institute for Biosocial Research has a complete library of books and tapes covering research that has been done using vitamins and amino acid therapy.

The *Clinical Journal of Nutrition* (January 1985) states that many patients with endogenous anxiety get an infusion of sodium lactate that can precipitate panic attacks. Glucose, which increases blood lactate levels, can also induce panic attacks in those who are susceptible. When stress is intensified, phobics have increased lactate levels, but they will improve greatly after large doses of vitamin B complex because B complex can lower levels of lactate. It is believed the action probably comes from niacinamide, thiamine, and pyridoxine factors in the B complex that convert lactate into pyruvic acid.

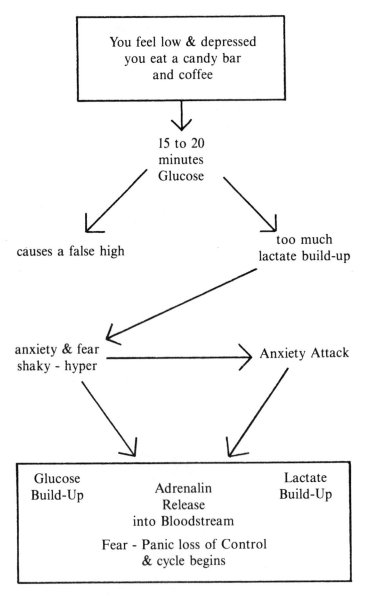

You feel low & depressed
you eat a candy bar
and coffee

15 to 20
minutes
Glucose

causes a false high

too much
lactate build-up

anxiety & fear
shaky - hyper

Anxiety Attack

Glucose
Build-Up

Adrenalin
Release
into Bloodstream

Lactate
Build-Up

Fear - Panic loss of Control
& cycle begins

*Lactate is a build-up of waste products
within the muscle, from
carbohydrate metabolism.*

The *Clinical Journal of Nutrition* advises patients with anxiety neurosis or agoraphobia to raise their intake of magnesium and B vitamins and eliminate caffeine and alcohol. Sugar and refined carbohydrates should be greatly reduced. Fructose converts rapidly into lactate; so does sorbitol and xylitol. Reading package contents and keeping track of daily intake could save the patient a lot of anxious times. Dr. Jeffrey Bland's statement that "you are what you absorb" becomes a statement of utmost importance to anxiety and phobia sufferers.

If you would like to see the effect of diet on your anxiety level, then eliminate caffeine, sugar, and alcohol for just one week. You will be pleased with your feeling of well being.

Bill Gottlieb wrote in *Prevention* magazine ("Nutrition: the Silver Lining," 1979) that many hyperactive children have low serotonin, tryptophan, and B6 levels. It appears that tryptophan raises the low levels of blood serotonin. Hyperactive children usually become hyperactive adults with anxiety. The deficiency from childhood is carried into adult life and, more importantly, if the children are sugarholics and consume caffeine in soft drinks they compound their own anxiety and panic just as do adults.

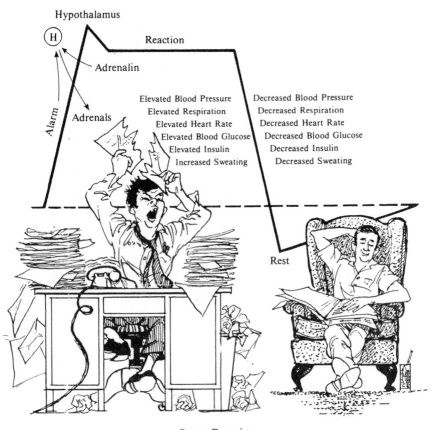

Hypothalamus

Reaction

Adrenalin

Alarm

Adrenals

Elevated Blood Pressure
Elevated Respiration
Elevated Heart Rate
Elevated Blood Glucose
Elevated Insulin
Increased Sweating

Decreased Blood Pressure
Decreased Respiration
Decreased Heart Rate
Decreased Blood Glucose
Decreased Insulin
Decreased Sweating

Rest

Stress Reaction

FEELINGS CYCLE

Anxiety is the fear of hurt or loss, nagging stress.

Hurt or *loss* leads to anger, anxiety, uncertainty.

Anger held in leads to guilt, depression, frustration.

Guilt unexpressed leads to depression.

Fear which is not confronted or understood becomes avoidance.

Avoidance of unresolved feelings leads to phobias.

Phobias lead to a constant control by overwhelming fear.

Fear leads to pain, physical and emotional.

Pain leads to fear, rational and irrational.

Uncertainty is nagging stress.

Repression is forcing a thought to the subconscious.

Frustration is loss of objectivity.

Dependency is need for a specific effect.

Resentment is mixed emotions, unsorted.

Awareness is acknowledgement of feelings.

Depersonalization is loss of identity.

Denial is refusal to admit reality.

Grief is the psychological and physical trauma state.

Sadness is the sense of a loss, and abnormal daily functioning.

VI
The Orthomolecular Approach to Treatment of Anxiety

In my work and research with people who suffer from anxiety, fear, panic, and phobias, one factor has surfaced continually: that anxiety has a direct effect on the body's physical/physiological symptoms.

In Dr. Harold Gelb's book, *Killing Pain Without a Prescription*, he stated that muscle tension causes most of the pain suffered in this country. Dr. Gelb showed that an astounding seventy to eighty million individuals suffer some type of muscular pain. Why? The precipitating factor in most cases is stress and their inability to cope with it.

Each of us begins to practice our coping skills as early as age four or five; the way in which we do or do not handle stress will be carried into our adult lives. Each person's ability to handle anxious/stressful situations depends on an extensive list of factors, including family environment, predispositions, child-parent relationships, and a lifelong challenge on stress conditioning, as well as our ability to be influenced by chronically ill or negative individuals around us. Factors that cause the damage are multiple, complex, and chronic.

Mechanized, Urbanized, Unbalanced Individual

Over-Rested Over-Fed Over-Stimulated
Over-Protected Under-Exercised Under-Released
Under-Disciplined

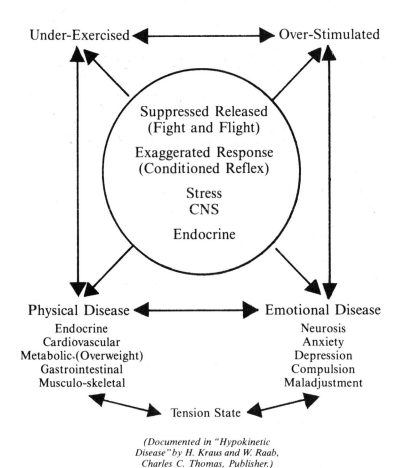

Under-Exercised ←———————→ Over-Stimulated

Suppressed Released
(Fight and Flight)

Exaggerated Response
(Conditioned Reflex)

Stress
CNS

Endocrine

Physical Disease ←———————→ Emotional Disease

Physical Disease	Emotional Disease
Endocrine	Neurosis
Cardiovascular	Anxiety
Metabolic (Overweight)	Depression
Gastrointestinal	Compulsion
Musculo-skeletal	Maladjustment

Tension State

*(Documented in "Hypokinetic
Disease" by H. Kraus and W. Raab,
Charles C. Thomas, Publisher.)*

ar of crowds, can't breathe
motional eating, food won't go down
uscle twitching
nable to remember
ithdrawal to home
ry cotton mouth
urred vision
ental confusion

r Natural Diet Supplement

ding to Roger J. Williams in *Nutrition Against*
n alcoholic should supplement his diet with a
tment of minerals and vitamins—even amino
e his years of drinking have typically caused
ment. A natural nutritional formula consists of
f vitamins, minerals, amino acids, and herbs to
lcoholic in his nutritional recovery. The formula
cal therapeutic replacement for toxic prescrip-
consists of the following substances.

CIDS

e the building blocks for our *proteins*. Proteins
l for a number of reasons:

ey furnish amino acids required for building of
ly tissues and health.
y supply food fuel for the body whenever in-
icient fats and carbohydrates are consumed;
y also help to maintain normal blood sugar.
ey assist in the transport of various minerals
l vitamins.
ey assist in the acid-base balance of the body.

n is needed for the health and formation of
ormones, membranes, glands, enzymes, skin,
eth, antibodies, ligaments, hair, fingernails,
ilage, hemoglobin, brain cells, and nerve cells.
and symptoms of insufficient protein intake
tigue, poor digestion, bloating, slow growth,
v vitality, sluggish pulse, scarring and slow heal-

An example of the situational anxiety that may develop from childhood to adulthood is the case of the offspring of an alcoholic such as Paul in Chapter II. Paul was exposed day in and day out to his father's illness and experienced loss of control, anxiety, fear, and a constant feeling of uncertainty. As a child and then as an adult, he suffered from a continuous anxious state. Imagine the condition of the chemoreceptors in his brain; is it not possible that the day-in day-out fearful state could damage or make the chemoreceptors oversensitive and so misfire? This—or traumatic occurrences of various kinds—would create panic from fear whenever flashbacks of his childhood occurred, especially if one or both parents were physically abusive.

Considering that alcoholics are malnourished, the condition of their children would probably not be average. Since every cell in our body changes completely every six months, it is what we are able to absorb that determines our state of health. If the alcoholic does not receive or is unable to absorb the necessary nutrients, essential amino acids, and minerals, he/she—and his/her child will stay in a minus state of nutrition predisposing them to both physical and emotional illnesses.

The tranquilizers which are so often given to alcoholics' children to help them cope and sleep are nothing more than a sugar coating or possibly the beginning of their own addiction. The tranquilizers simply cover up the symptoms, but do not remove the cause.

In *Brain Allergies—The Psychonutrient Connection*, by William H. Philpott, M.D., and Dwight Kalita, Ph.D., the authors state that toximolecular psychiatrists (those who use drugs or synthetic substances not normally found in the human body) may think they are practicing scientific medicine, but they are not. Even though tranquilizers manage to control psychiatric symptoms, the underlying disease process initially responsible for the symptom usually remains unchecked.

Linus Pauling in defining "orthomolecular medicine" said that the treatment of disease is a matter of "varying the concentration of substances (i.e., the right molecules:

vitamins, minerals, trace elements, hormones, amino acids, enzymes) normally present in the human body." Through regulation of the concentration of chemical molecules, orthomolecular medicine aims at the achievement and preservation of optimum health and the prevention and treatment of disease.

Many physicians are unfamiliar with the orthomolecular approach and know only the drug or toximolecular approach. Dr. Philpott states that "drugs are chemical substances which, even if given singly, radically alter man's metabolic machinery and many times interfere with normal vitamin, mineral, amino-acids and enzyme activities in the body. Nutrients, on the other hand, working as a team, act constructively as building blocks for life in general; without them, human life could not exist. Life can exist without drugs!"

Abram Hoffer, M.D., Ph.D., an orthomolecular psychiatrist, has warned that he has seen many hyperactive young children that were placed on symptomatic drug therapy such as Ritalin. This type of therapy brings hyperactive symptoms emotionally under control, but later the patient degenerates further into adult schizophrenia; the adult schizophrenia results because the underlying metabolic cause remains untreated.

Toximolecular medicine requires only one thing from its patients—that they continue to take their drugs or tranquilizers. It is disturbing to think that these patients on drugs often have to pay an extremely high price for their symptomatic relief; they run the statistically high risk of becoming permanently incarcerated and/or controlled by their chemical straitjackets.

Hoffer and Walker in *Orthomolecular Nutrition* offer the following summary:

> Every tissue of the body is affected by nutrition. Under conditions of poor nutrition the kidney stops filtering, the stomach stops digesting, the adrenals stop secreting, and other organs follow suit. Unfortunately, some psychiatrists labor under the false belief that somehow brain func-

tion is completely
seems that many psy
chiatric colleagues
social workers consi
of the body that nee

I repeat once more—
quilizer deficiency.

Symptoms of Anxiety

The following are s
phobia symptoms that l
orthomolecular therapy:

1. Feeling a loss of
2. Going insane
3. Light-headednes
4. Unsteady legs
5. Difficulty in bre breath
6. Fear of heart att
7. Heart pounding,
8. Constant fear of
9. Tingling lips and
10. Stomach pain, d bottomlessness
11. Excessive sweatin
12. Headaches, neck
13. Low back pain
14. Tender-headednes
15. Feeling tired, wea
16. Feeling as though
17. Mood and emotio
18. Unable to sleep
19. Restless sleep; nig
20. Unable to relax
21. Anxiety, tension, r
22. Depressing or neg
23. Need to have som
24. Rush of panic or f

25.
26.
27.
28.
29.
30.
31.
32.

Formula

Acc
Disease,
good ass
acids," s
malnouri
a number
assist the
of this ty
tion dru

AMINO

These
are esser

1.
2.
3.
4.

Pro
muscles
plasma,
bones, c
Sig
include:
anemia,

ing, frequent infections, fragile bones, wrinkled skin, senility, dental caries, weakness, and abnormal blood pressure.

DLPA (*DL-phenylalanine*) is one of the essential amino acids. It has been found helpful in the control of depression and pain. Our bodies produce their own morphine-like substances in the brain called endorphins; one form of the endorphin is 500 times more powerful than morphine. Unfortunately, we have enzymes in the body which break down the endorphin very rapidly before we really obtain the benefit of it. The DLPA slows the action of the enzyme so that we are able to derive benefits from the endorphin.

GABA (*Gamma-aminobutyric acid*) is an amino acid complex which, when taken with niacinamide and inositol, calms anxiety and stress reactions. The GABA receptors in the brain are the sites where drugs like Valium, Librium, and Ativan act.

L-tyrosine is the first breakdown of phenylalanine in the liver. Tyrosine is an amino acid that is helpful in overcoming depression. Clinical studies have shown that L-tyrosine controls medication-resistant depression. In 1980, in the *American Journal of Psychiatry*, a study by Dr. Alan Gelenberg of the Department of Psychiatry at Harvard Medical School discussed the role of L-tyrosine in the control of anxiety and depression. Dr. Gelenberg postulated that a lack of available L-tyrosine results in a deficiency of the hormone norepinephrine at a specific brain location, which, in turn, relates to mood problems, such as depression.

Alcohol shares many similar properties with the hypnotic and anti-anxiety drugs. Alcohol seems to serve as courage for the alcoholic since it seems to work primarily on anticipatory anxiety. The alcoholic is in a state of chronic anxiety. As a side note, alcohol has been shown to operate as a MAO inhibitor.*

---

*MAO, or monomine oxidase, is an enzyme which can oxidize —and thus deactivate—various aminos, including serotonin, the catecholamines and their methoxy derivatives. A MAO inhibitor is a category of antidepressant.

Glutamine is one of the twelve non-essential amino acids. (Non-essential simply means that, given the substances needed, the body can manufacture the amino acid.) Dr. Roger Williams at the Clayton Foundation for Research at the University of Texas has done extensive research in L-glutamine. Dr. William Shive discovered that L-glutamine protected bacteria cells against the poisoning by alcohol. In addition, it was discovered by Dr. Lorene Rogers that L-glutamine stopped the craving for alcohol. L-glutamine becomes glutamic acid in the brain and increases the amount of GABA.

B AND C—THE WATER SOLUBLE VITAMINS

Vitamin B is actually a "complex" of several vitamins. These include B1-thiamine, B2-riboflavin, B3-niacin (niacinamide), B6-pyridoxine, B12, pantothenic acid (calcium pantothenate), biotin, PABA (para-aminobenzoic acid), folic acid, choline, and inositol. All the B1 vitamins are water soluble and are excreted via the kidneys in the urine. They are not stored in the body and therefore must be supplied in sufficient amounts at all times—especially when the body is under stress of any kind.

Even though the B vitamins are supplied in the diet in quantities to support normal health, this can be inadequate under stress unless the "B's" are supplied in good amounts. *Stress* is anything that causes extra tension—emotional and/or physical—on the body; for example: drugs, alcohol, chemicals, excessive fatigue, noise, infections, emotional turmoil, anxiety. Recall that alcohol is a source of energy (calories) in the body; alcohol is definitely a carbohydrate and is broken down to sugar in the body. The B vitamins are required in the burning of alcohol in the body; if large amounts of carbohydrates are consumed, the individual should also increase his daily intake of the B vitamins.

Ascorbic acid—Vitamin C is water soluble and is excreted via the kidneys in the urine and skin in perspiration. Vitamin C is essential to the body for the formation of collagen in the body; collagen is a protein substance that cements together the cells of the body to make tissue. Collagen is important to the body for the following reasons:

1. It is necessary for the development of health capillaries, bones, cartilage, teeth, and connective tissue.
2. It is important in protecting the body from infection.
3. It aids the adrenal production of cortisone.
4. It assists in the absorption of iron from the intestines.

Vitamin C is an anti-oxidant; it helps to neutralize foreign substances, chemicals, and poisons in the body. The body's need for Vitamin C increases greatly during times of stress; again, this is *any* form of stress—emotional, environmental, physical, or during infections.

Scurvy is the most severe deficiency of a lack of vitamin C; this is fairly rare in the United States today. However, many signs and symptoms of mild to moderate deficiencies are seen which include the following: dental caries, bleeding gums, gum disease, tendency to bruise easily, inclination toward sinus problems, allergies, and hayfever, and greater incidence of viral and bacterial infections.

A, D, E—THE FAT SOLUBLE VITAMINS

Vitamin A is a fat-soluble vitamin, i.e., the presence of fat is necessary in the diet for vitamin A to be properly absorbed by the intestines. Chronic alcohol ingestion may result in the liver's decreased ability to store vitamin A in the liver, actually leading to a deficiency.

Vitamin D, the sunshine vitamin, is also a member of the fat-soluble vitamin family. Exposure of the skin to the sunshine produces vitamin D which is then absorbed into the body. The primary place of storage is in the liver. It is necessary for the body to properly utilize calcium and phosphorus which is important for strong bones and teeth.

Vitamin E is also a fat-soluble vitamin; its absorption may be limited in anyone having fat metabolism disturbances such as an alcoholic might have after many years of drinking. Vitamin E's most important function is that of an anti-oxidant; this is especially important to the alcoholic. It also plays a role in the protection of vitamin A as well as fats and oils.

THE MINERALS

While minerals comprise only 4 to 5 percent of the body's total weight, these "elements" are very powerful substances. Vitamins *cannot* function without the assistance of the minerals. Minerals work together as a group, rather than individually. They work in conjunction with hormones, enzymes, proteins, amino acids, carbohydrates, fats, and vitamins. They are required for the proper overall mental and physical functioning of the body and help to build and maintain the body structure.

Calcium is the most abundant mineral found in the body. While 99% of the calcium is found in bones and teeth, the other 1% is in the soft tissues and blood; this 1% has great effect on the nerves. A double-blind study with anxiety-prone patients and normal patients showed strong similarities between the symptoms of an anxiety attack and the mental effects of calcium deficiency, thus giving further evidence of the importance of calcium in mental health.

Magnesium is an important mineral. It is a natural tranquilizer for the nervous system. Magnesium is required for protein and for carbohydrate metabolism. Signs of magnesium deficiency are similar to common hangover symptoms: sensitivity to noise, tremors, twitching, dizziness, rapid heartbeat, aching muscles, fatigue, depression, and irritability. Magnesium has been used in treating anxiety, depression, and insomnia. In mental function, magnesium is the *only* electrolyte which has a higher level in the brain fluid than in the blood plasma.*

Potassium is vital for the proper functioning of nerves,

---

*Electrolyte is a solution which is a conductor of electricity, or a substance which, in solution, conducts an electrical current and is decomposed by the passage of an electric current. Acids, bases, and salts are common electrolytes.

heart, and muscles; in addition, it works with sodium to maintain the body's water/salt balance. Potassium deficiency symptoms include muscular fatigue, lack of appetite, and mental apathy. Hypoglycemia (low blood sugar) causes a loss of potassium; hypoglycemia seems to be present in many alcoholics.

Phosphorus is important in nearly all physiological chemical reactions; it is necessary for normal bone and teeth structure and for the transmission of nerve impulses. Phosphorus aids in body repairs, and is helpful in the metabolization of fats and starches.

Manganese is found throughout the body, but especially the liver, skin, bones, and muscles. It is necessary for the proper digestion and utilization of food; manganese is important for normal central nervous system function. It helps eliminate fatigue and reduces nervous irritability.

Iron is an important mineral since over half of the body's iron is found in the red blood cells as part of the hemoglobin, and hemoglobin is the protein that carries oxygen to the body tissues. The amino acids in protein, vitamin C, and copper all enhance the absorption of iron.

Zinc, last but not least, is involved in many enzyme systems with a wide scope of actions. Zinc and vitamin A work as a pair—vitamin A is mobilized from the liver by zinc. After the ingestion of alcohol or large amounts of drugs, zinc is excreted in the urine in large amounts; many alcoholics are zinc deficient. This deficiency actually increases the alcoholic's tolerance to liquor, for there is a strong reaction to alcohol when the body contains adequate quantities of zinc. The drinker who "can hold his liquor" does not have as much zinc—and is not as healthy —as the person who gets drunk with one drink. Other signs of zinc deficiency include oily skin, hair loss, lack of appetite, loss of taste, apathy, and lethargy.

Others. The remaining minerals—sodium, sulfur, chlorine, and fluorine—are also essential minerals, but of less importance than those above.

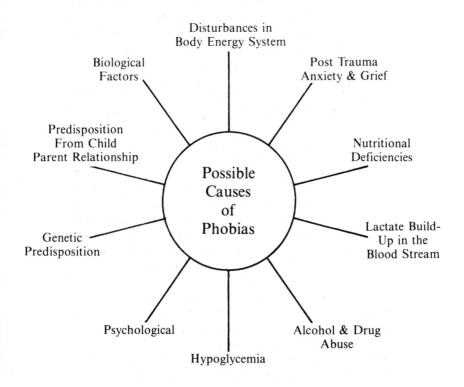

VII
Solving the Puzzle
—The Healing Begins

Empathetic Understanding—This kind
of understanding is sharply different from
the usual evaluative understanding,
which follows the pattern of, "I understand
what is wrong with you." When there
is a sensitive empathy, however, the reaction
in the learner follows something of this
pattern: "At last someone understands how
it feels and seems to be me, without
wanting to analyze or judge me. Now I can
blossom and grow and learn." This is
the very special way of being with another
person which is called "empathetic."

Carl Rogers
A Way of Being

Dr. Rogers sums up what I consider the most important
factor in reaching and helping a person who has suffered
for many years. A therapist's own empathy is his best
qualification. Through this process he is able to put a face
on the patient's fear for the first time and light up a part of
the sufferer's life that has been shrouded in dread and
darkness. Empathy creates a bond between the therapist

and the patient, especially when the therapist does not identify himself as an authority figure or become judgemental. That special empathy is part of a *wounded healer* —one who has suffered and walked from the face of fear and darkness to light and understanding. Choose one who walks *with* you, not in front of you.

Dr. Rogers demonstrates the potential for success in reaching out. "When the other person is hurting, confused, troubled, anxious, alienated, terrified, or when he or she is doubtful of self-worth, uncertain as to identity . . . then understanding is called for. The gentle and sensitive compassion offered by an empathetic person provides illumination and healing. In such situations deep understanding and sharing is, I believe, the most precious gift one can give another."

Implementing a Multi-Dimensional Approach to Desensitization and Healing

A large part of moving through your anxiety, fear, and phobias is to accept responsibility for *yourself and only yourself.* This means choosing, making hard decisions, accepting consequences, getting rid of excuses, and blaming no one; and, too, exploring all natural resources for mind and body—listening to and becoming aware of your body's needs, as well as its rejections.

The subconscious can handle only so much storing of the negative, only so many times that you say, "I can't handle that . . . I can't deal with that." There comes a time for dealing, and if you don't stop and deal with it now, when will you deal with it? When a person lacks the capacity to act on the basis of their own power, they are setting themselves up to be threatened by every new situation which requires autonomous action.

Another strong factor enters the picture . . . *repression*. Repression of needs, true feelings, anger, and self-esteem. Repression decreases autonomy and increases helplessness and inner conflict.

Anxiety and hostility are interrelated—one generates the other. First, anxiety gives rise to hostility. This can be understood in its simplest form in the fact that anxiety, mixed with hostility, creates helpless isolation, and conflict —all become exceedingly powerful experiences.

Other powerful and painful emotions must deal with the loss of self-esteem, loss of confidence, and the feeling that you can't do anything right. All of those things depend on you, *your* judgement. Whatever your own concept of anxiety is, it is just that—it is your own concept. Anxiety as well as fear and phobias are all your own, they are unique to you, and they all have your own personal characteristics. Anxiety reflects the kind of personality you have developed from infancy and childhood through your adult life right up to today.

At times, in childhood as well as maturity, when anxiety cannot find a way to release, it surfaces in physical form. The result may be an outbreak of hives, a migraine headache, or neck pain, or even sudden weight gain or loss. "Arthur" came to me twenty-four hours after an outbreak of hives caused by an anxiety attack. He felt helpless, but he was repressing these emotions. He did not see the relationship between the anxiety and the hives.

Anxiety, stress, fear, and pain will always attack your weak spots, and they know where they are—migraines, stomach, back, headaches, sweating, nightmares. Don't fight it, understand it. Deal with it for what it is . . . an emotional outpouring. To give in to it or to refuse to see what it is trying to point out is to let it become much stronger and gain that much more control.

Acknowledge the panic, the anxiety, then sort it out and look at it. Take the positive, take the negative, and examine it from both sides. It can't grow if you are sorting it out . . . if you are dealing with it, if you are in touch with it. "I know what's happening," you tell yourself, "I know what's going on."

Confront fear, confront anxiety. "Why am I afraid of the situation? What do I think is going to happen? . . . What am I anticipating? . . . What has happened in the past that I think is going to happen now? Why do I feel I have no control?"

Relax, let time pass; don't hyperventilate. Understand what is going on inside of you. Remember, *a relaxed muscle cannot have an anxiety attack—it is impossible.*

Don't run, let your feelings come, don't fight the feelings of panic. When you feel the panic mount, relax, take a deep breath, always inhaling through your nose and exhaling slowly through your mouth. Reinforce: "Nothing is going to happen! I'm okay!"

The reality within you is a great asset and your conscious mind is only waiting for you to say, "Wait a minute, I'm going to bring this thing into perspective." Maybe you can't drive on the expressway right now, but the longer you sit there and think about it, the more fearful you become. Negative thinking produces negative action.

In helping phobics work through panic and anxiety, I have found that teaching them self-hypnosis is very effective. Since all hypnosis is self-hypnosis, or an altered state consciousness, you can use it to project yourself through fearful situations and remain relaxed.

The easiest way to get into an altered state is to take a few slow, deep breaths, let your eyes close, and count slowly from ten to one. When you open your eyes you will be completely relaxed. (See Self-Help chapter for procedure.) With practice you can use the self-hypnosis to work through many difficult situations. When I learned this procedure, it became one of my main keys to conquer fear. The more I would go through it in my mind the less anxious I would become.

As a practical example—I use it today when I go to the dentist. In the past, I had had an unpleasant experience when a dentist almost let me gag on cotton, and it left me with a fear of choking. I told my new dentist of the episode, and he helped me overcome this irrational fear. When I learned the technique of self-hypnosis, I decided to avoid the hanging lower lip which results from a shot of Novacaine, and learned to put myself into a deep state and feel no pain. The system is easier on me and on the dentist. Now I send him many anxious and fearful patients, and he is wonderfully successful with them.

Projecting yourself successfully through a situation reinforces the assurance that nothing will happen. The anxiety only last for minutes; control comes with your ability to relax and remain relaxed. Fear and relaxation don't mix. And each successful experience makes the next easier to achieve.

Let me go over again a few constructive ways in which you can handle anxiety—instead of its handling you. The key is an expansion of awareness. Don't let the conflict get started. Restructure your goals if you have to, make allowances if needed, but don't give in and be unrealistic and say "I can't do it." *You* are the one in control. You achieve what you believe you can achieve. You achieve what you want to achieve. And when you have achieved something, the feeling within you is projected, and what is projected becomes the confidence and the self-esteem that you need to overcome the anxious feelings.

These are all therapeutic ways of dealing with yourself, a self you can continue to improve or a self that you can allow to become stagnant. Your life is yours. You need not be controlled by fear. People talk about someone hearing a different drummer . . . you may not feel the same way somebody else does about a situation . . . that's OK. You have a right to feel differently.

Create your own mountain, and when you get to the top of that mountain you will not find any anxiety or fear. Leave the chronic apprehensiveness at the bottom as you climb. It doesn't matter if the mountain is very small in the beginning . . . each time you climb it it will become bigger and you will become stronger. As your growth continues, so will your happiness. Growth and happiness increase one's awareness; use it to reduce anxiety and fear to normal levels and then use the normal anxiety to stimulate your own awareness.

Another way of saying it is that anxiety is a signal that something is wrong in one's personality or relationships. You may view anxiety as an inward cry for resolution—resolution of a problem that you've been carrying . . . unresolved anxiety. The cause, of course, can have an infinite number of sources.

It may be the result of some misunderstanding between you and your mother or father, or with a friend, lover, or spouse, which can be resolved with authentic *communication* with the other person. Open communication can resolve a surprising number of problematic or frightening situations. It is our refusal to communicate ... our fear to communicate . . . our lack of knowledge of how to communicate . . . our fear of telling someone how we feel so that they can better deal with us and we can deal with ourselves and others—*that* is the basis of our relationship problems.

Or perhaps what is wrong is some expectation of one's self at a stage of development when it cannot be realistically achieved, and that is very important. If you feel that you are not able to accomplish what you should, then you become anxious and may go into avoidance. Anxiety may be triggered by an awareness of the limitations of your life —limitations of one's intelligence, relationships, unavoidable loneliness, or some other aspect of one's life. In these cases, anxiety may take the form of mild or great dread.

The intensity of these situations can, of course, vary. Dread may be simple undercurrents of apprehension, or graphic imagining of something about to happen to us. In these cases, we tend to use a tremendous amount of negative thinking to deal with the fear or we go into complete avoidance and perhaps even become housebound. This is our way of not confronting—of refusing to face the problem.

One of the most thoroughly phobic patients I have ever worked with was "Sister Karen," a fifty-one-year-old nun who was a high school teacher and counselor. She was an introvert, a workaholic, and an agoraphobiac. She began to develop phobias as she continued to internalize her anger, fear, and depression. There were several bouts of physical illness due to extreme fatigue—both physical and mental. She had been hurt emotionally numerous times and was never able to deal with it. Her anxiety began to deepen and the phobic physical symptoms continued to take control.

Here is the incredible list of fears she presented at a session:

1. Fear of death
2. Fear to let others know what's happening inside of me
3. Fear of not being accepted
4. Fear of being useless
5. Fear of being dependent
6. Fear of being incapacitated
7. Fear of going blind
8. Fear of what others think about me
9. Fear of being in an accident
10. Fear of being late
11. Fear of knowing who I really am
12. Fear of not being strong enough
13. Fear of not being able to handle family death
14. Fear of what may happen to my brother in his marriage
15. Fear of my oldest sister
16. Fear of authority
17. Fear of hurting others
18. Fear of appearing before a large group
19. Fear of giving my opinion
20. Fear that my way of sharing may be all off target, or that I do not explain myself intelligently
21. Fear when someone calls me aside to say something
22. Fear at times when called to the phone
23. Fear of becoming very weak and collapsing somewhere
24. Fear of going out of my mind
25. Fear of being in a psycho ward
26. Fear of not leaving another free—of getting in their way
27. Fear lest people will not be/are not open and honest with me
28. Fear of not doing a good job
29. Fear of being in church (in a large crowd) for a long service; needing to sit on the end of a bench
30. Fear of the future
31. Fear of losing my vocation
32. Fear of people not keeping my confidences.

The first step in helping this woman was reality therapy—and getting her to relax and let her feelings out. She needed reassurance that it was OK to say, do, or be whatever she felt. She had a tremendous fear of drugs or any type loss of control.

A nutritional evaluation proved that she was physically depleted to a dangerous degree. Nutritional supplements were suggested and this proved to be very beneficial.

After six months of therapy, Sister Karen began to recover and her personality-strengths came to the surface. Now she knows who, what, or how—it's OK to be who you are. I cannot help feeling that a major influence in this case was the fact that I could understand the depth of her pain because I had once walked the same paths, felt the deep hurt and wondered what the Lord had in store for me. It had come to me finally that my purpose was to give of myself, to help others but not to lose my identity.

Sister Karen has been sent down the same path. Watching her become enriched by life has reinforced my convictions of why I am on this earth. Today Sister Karen is like no other and her presence is known and felt by all others in a positive beauty that radiates when she enters a room.

Understand Your Body Biochemistry

An ordinary day of physical exercise is a pleasant experience which puts you in a happy mood. The epinephrine (adrenaline) that goes to your heart is normal. But when you are in a situation of extreme anxiety or panic, the increase in the amount of adrenaline, plus sudden infusion of more hormones knows as catecholamines (adrenaline), can disrupt the rhythm of the heart. If the constant stress on the heart continues it could rupture the heart muscle fibers.

If you are relaxed and without anxiety and fear, you will be able to do whatever you enjoy. The power of the mind (projecting calm, relaxed, and at peace), such as in self-hypnosis, programs the brain and hormones and endocrine system. You are your own protector. Uncertainty is the number one situation which causes anxiety to become a panic state.

Uncertainty ➜ Anxiety ➜ Panic ➜ Fear ➜ Phobia

Biofeedback Therapy

Biofeedback training is an excellent way to mirror the changes in your body. This information tells you what physical changes are happening to you under stress. With biofeedback training you are able to learn how to slow down your heart and realize what a state of total relaxation is—in contrast to an anxiety attack.

Biofeedback is the use of instrumentation to mirror psychophysiological processes of which the individual is not normally aware and which may be brought under voluntary control. This means giving the subject immediate information about his own biological conditions, such as muscle tension, skin surface temperature, brain wave activity, galvanic skin response, blood rate, and heart rate. This feedback enables the individual to become an active participant in the process of phobic desensitization.

Biofeedback involves the use of specialized instrumentation. The equipment may be as simple as a thermometer or as sophisticated as an electroencephalograph —an electronic device which measures brain wave patterns. The most important feature about the instrumentation, no matter how simple or complex, is that it tells the individual about the measurement which it has just made. It is this important feature of measurement and immediate report which distinguishes biofeedback from other techniques that teach "relaxation" or "alpha control," but which do not involve feedback of actual physiological changes.

Hold a small thermometer between your finger and thumb, and think about your fear. Your temperature will drop and your hands will become cold. Now begin to breathe deeply and slowly and let go of the fear, and watch your temperature rise. That is how fast your body records change of fear and anxiety. Self-hypnosis with biofeedback is one of the best ways to train yourself to control stress and anxiety.

The use of biofeedback instrumentation is merely a means to an end. It is a very useful learning technique whereby the individual can learn better control over certain psychophysiological processes. The end result is that you can exercise this voluntary control without the use of any instruments. Your major goal is to learn to lower muscle tension, anxiety level, and panic. Biofeedback training is well worth your time and effort. It is something you will use in many situations and for years to come. Anxiety cannot be completely avoided but it can be reduced. The problem of management of anxiety is that of reducing the anxiety to normal levels and then using the normal anxiety as stimulation to increase one's awareness.

Stress and anxiety cause us to put our body in a deficient state. Understanding your nutritional strengths and weaknesses is extremely important, but don't go out and buy a quantity of vitamins and "megadose." It won't do you any good, and it will be a waste of good money. Locate an orthomolecular physician, therapist, or nutritionist, and get a complete work-up. (Do not use hair analysis. Hair analysis was termed inaccurate according to the Texas Medical Association in November 1983.)

Once you have established your nutritional needs, don't expect miracles. You've had the deficiencies for a while and it takes time to rebuild your system.

The amino acids therapy outlined in this book is used by orthomolecular physicians. There are two products on the market now for anxiety sufferers, one for adults and one for children. The stress and anxiety formula contains both GABA and tyrosine, which I have described in detail in previous chapters. I personally use this formula at stressful times, when my anxiety is high, and it works for me. There is a special product for children which contains GABA and tryptophan and addresses children's deficiencies as I have described.*

---

*For further information, write to The Pain & Stress Center in San Antonio, Texas.

VIII
The Self-Help Movement

The doctor of the future
will give no medicine
but will interest his patients
in the care of the human frame,
in diet, and in the cause and
prevention of disease.
Thomas A. Edison

The first time I saw a self-help magazine I was extremely happy—to say the least—that publishers were aware there was a need for this information. Then, month by month, more and more began to appear.

In 1976, I saw a report on L-tryptophan, the natural relaxant. I focused on "natural" and "relaxant" and realized there was an alternative to drugs and that many others were seeking the same thing. Searching for the new product at drugstores proved fruitless until finally one pharmacist suggested that a health food store should have L-tryptophan. They did. I slept better that night than I had in a long time. Then my search for information about amino acids began—and still goes on today.

The forerunners in the research in the U.S. were Drs.

Kenneth Pelletier and David Bresler whose work in the field of psychosomatic pain opened many doors. In 1978, Dr. Pelletier released a cassette tape, "Mental Stress—Physical Symptoms," which sold 3½ to 4 million copies in the first year. Its contents give a clear, concise picture of the power of the mind and how, as our stress level goes up, our painful physical symptoms continue to occur until we cannot function.

Dr. Bresler, then director of UCLA Pain Control Unit, issued a tape on chronic pain and alternatives to drugs. In his book "Free Yourself from Pain," Dr. Bresler covers the use of amino acids, especially studies of tryptophan.

In 1980, Marilyn Ferguson published *The Aquarian Conspiracy*, which became a non-fiction topseller. This book talked about the personal and social transformation in the 80's. Under her section on "Healing Ourselves," she defines psychiatry as literally "doctoring the soul." It is unlikely that great doses of tranquilizing drugs can heal a fractured soul; rather, they interrupt the pattern of distress and conflict by altering the brain's disturbed chemistry.

It may take a bit more time for the medical profession as a whole to accept the new concept of holistic healing in general and non-drug treatment of stress and pain in particular, but as the information is brought to public attention the change will come. As patients realize that there are alternatives to the usual rounds of toxic prescriptions to achieve freedom from pain, they will request safer products and other treatments.

The integral approach is a new focus emerging within the health care community today; it is characterized by an integrated approach to the patient or individual. Rather than treatment of the individual parts, the treatment is centered around the "whole" person. Emphasis is placed on the psychological parts of the healing process, and the importance of maintaining health and wellness instead of the treatment of disease. Clinicians and research scientists are now investigating radical new procedures and techniques which hold the promise for a longer life and better health. As a result, therapeutic techniques once considered eccentric are being accepted by the public and the medical community. For example, acupuncture, yoga, herbology, homeopathy, hypnosis, guided imagery, and biofeedback are now being sought out by a health-conscious public. In the treatment of psychosomatic and psychosocial diseases of civilization, a variety of nonsomatic factors must be carefully examined. Such conditions as the inability to handle stress, a loss, or an adjustment effectively, problems in family or work environments, belief and expectations, having feelings of no control over your life, self-destructive habits, and a host of problems connected to human sexuality—are all known to affect the onset of the illness and the outcome of the therapy. The enormous power of the mind has just begun to be explored. It seems apparent that a combination of mental, spiritual, and physical approaches can help to implement the body's intrinsic healing powers and ability for self-regulation in ways previously thought impossible. Further research may yield even more innovative techniques for creating and maintaining health.

Practitioners of integral medicine are concerned mainly with an individual rather than a disease. They view the universal life force as a benevolent process that stimulates and supports human development. Symptoms are viewed as a warning that something is wrong. The meaning of illness is explored through a therapeutic partnership in which patients and clinicians exchange information, advice, and support.

Integral medicine utilizes some aspects of holistic medicine, and it also uses "traditional" medicine. Integral medicine practitioners use individual combinations of both traditional and nontraditional approaches which places most of the responsibility with the patient in the treatment process. Through the utilization and integration of both the old and new methods of practice into the existing health care delivery system, the patient is offered comprehensive care and may be helped where he may not have been helped by symptomatic therapy. As a result, both the patients and their doctors are rediscovering the mutual trust and confidence that has traditionally been characteristic of the doctor-patient relationship.

The trend toward specialization is becoming more

equilibrated by the search for an integrated understanding of the life process; old rituals and new technologies are being brought together in unique and innovative ways. As a result, in the process both are altered and the potential for total patient care is nearer to becoming a reality.

For example, for a patient who has injured his back, *traditional* medicine would base treatment on drugs and surgery. *Holistic* medicine would focus on noninvasive alternative approaches. *Integral* medicine would draw from either or both and choose the best therapy for the individual needs of the patient. Further, traditional medicine believes that disease is caused primarily by physical factors and holistic medicine emphasizes the mental, emotional, and social factors which are to blame; integral medicine sees disease as a multifaceted process which results from an interaction of all these factors, each assuming different responsibilities.

This will be the medicine of the future and I thoroughly believe that the use of GABA is exciting and has a profound effect on the psychological as well as the physical feelings of the patient. In order to achieve the integral effect, other forms of therapy such as laser and electro-acuscope, nutritional counseling, therapeutic massage, biofeedback and homeopathy, hypnosis and herbology—taking the best of two worlds—must not be overlooked. So that in the end the person who benefits is the *patient*.

Throughout this book I have discussed drastic change in the way people view medicine and their growing awareness of the natural products such as GABA, tryptophan, DL-phenylalanine, glutamine, and other important nutrients which are available to replace painkillers and antidepressants. If it were not for the pioneer in the field, Dr. Kenneth Pelletier, Director of the Institute of Psychosomatic Medicine in San Francisco, we might not be as far ahead at this point as we are now.

During the years 1975-76, any time the term "psychosomatic" was applied to a physical symptom, even physicians would turn away and avoid discussion of treatment for the patient. The strongest support for the validity of the term came from Dr. Pelletier's first book, *Mind as Healer*,

Mind as Slayer, where he emphatically defined psychosomatic medicine. At that point, 90% of the American public thought that a diagnosis of an illness as psychosomatic in nature meant that their pain was imaginary or that they were crazy or that they had some type of emotional illness. Dr. Pelletier often refers to the "internist's bible," Harrison's *Principles of Internal Medicine*, which states that 50 to 80 percent of all disease is psychosomatic in nature. From this basis, he has defined psychosomatic illness as we know it today.

Psychosomatic illness does not mean that the patient has an emotional illness, nor that the pain is imaginary; the pain is real and the patient is indeed suffering—even more so than with organic pathology. Pelletier emphatically went on record and named many of the illnesses which were being treated by all phases of medicine (ranging from peptic ulcers, migraines, ulcerated colitis, bronchial asthma, muscle spasms, and hayfever to Reynaud's disease, hypertension, hyperthyroidism, rheumatoid arthritis, myosistis, and edema) and he stated that these are stress-induced symptoms and that they are, in fact, psychosomatic in nature and have no pathology. It was during these years, 1975-80, that Drs. Pelletier, David Bresler, and Martin Rossman began the campaign to inform and educate the public as to the meaning of stress and anxiety-induced psychosomatic illness, and to teach them that not all psychosomatic illness requires traditional drugs.

The integral medicine approach was developed and implemented into a program for healthcare practitioners through UCLA Medical School. The founder and director of the Integral Medicine Program was Dr. Bresler. Other practitioners were Norman Shealy, M.D., Ph.D., Director of the Shealy Pain Clinic; Ronald Katz, M.D., Dennis Jaffe, Ph.D., Nancy Solomon, M.D., and Carl Simonton, M.D. In addition, pioneering clinicians and research scientists are now seriously investigating radically new techniques that hold the promise of longer life and better health. As a result, therapeutic procedures once considered eccentric or esoteric are receiving increasing public acceptance and scientific validation.

IX
Self-Help
Information

The information in this chapter will help you help yourself in handling anxiety and its causes and effects. Following are procedures, materials, and suggestions which can be of use to you.

Self-Hypnosis or Autogenic Training

If your fear is caused by stress or anxiety, this exercise will help you release it in just a few minutes:

Find a comfortable spot where you can be alone and it is quiet and without any bright lights. Close your eyes and take a very . . . deep . . . slow . . . abdominal breath. As you exhale, imagine that you're holding a leaf in the air and watch it fall gently to the earth. And each time you inhale and exhale, bring another leaf gently down to earth.

Continue to breathe very deeply and very slowly, and imagine, if you'd like, that your body has just been surrounded by a warm, soft blanket. Let go . . . allow the tension to flow out.

Maybe you'd like to walk along the beach, smell the salt air, and feel the warm wind. Maybe you'd like to be all alone in a big forest and sit under a big tree and watch the leaves fall. Maybe you'd like to be on the top of a snow-covered mountain where the only sound you hear is the crunch of snow under your feet.

Go wherever you want to, but as you do, let your stress go. Feel each one of your muscles beginning to relax . . . feeling very warm . . . very heavy. Maybe you'd like to walk by a small creek. Maybe your favorite place is high in the sky. Wherever it is, spend a brief few minutes releasing all of the stress and pain . . . letting it flow out . . . feeling warm . . . relaxed . . . calm . . . breathing deeply . . . slowly. It doesn't take long, once you allow your body to let go. You'll notice as you continue breathing slowly and deeply . . . that parts of your body will begin to tingle. The more relaxed they are, the less tense they are.

Perhaps you would like to just be in your favorite chair at home, or sitting in the middle of a big field. You can visualize any one of these places and in just a few minutes you'll notice that your whole body feels very warm . . . very loose. You can do this exercise several times a day. If you can't get away from your office, just close your eyes and give your body a signal breath and tell it that it has permission to relax those tense muscles and wrap itself in the warm blanket and let all of the pain drain out . . . and feel it leave your body.

Pre-set a number—"by the time I count to seven I will be completely and totally relaxed." Then you can give your body a signal by beginning to count, and by the time you reach seven . . . breathing very deeply and slowly . . . all of your muscles will be like warm, soft sand. Try to repeat this exercise as often as you can . . . at lunch, or in the middle of the afternoon.

This is one simple way to let your fear and stress drift away.

Self-Programming Stress Control

Your mind is still . . .
if you have any last thoughts or worries
watch them float away
like small clouds in a calm, blue sky . . .
you are at peace . . .

You are completely at peace . . .
Relax and enjoy the sunlight
Relax and enjoy the breeze . . .
Relax . . . Float . . . Drift.
Breathe gently and deeply . . .
        and relax . . .
Your body is rested and at peace.

You are calm . . .
Rested . . . Safe . . . Peaceful.
Relax and feel your tension
        drift away.
Relax . . . Float . . . Drift.
You are at Peace . . .
You are as one.

Use self-programming at least twice a day—or at any time you feel stressful. Use deep breathing as you repeat the words to yourself.

BRAIN PATHWAYS OF MENTAL DISTRESS

Anxiety and Alcohol

The neurotransmitter GABA normally modulates anxiety in the brain. Intoxication strongly affects processes controlled areas with high concentrations of GABA receptors, including motor coordination (cerebellum), information retrieval (hippocampus) and cognitive processes (cerebral cortex).

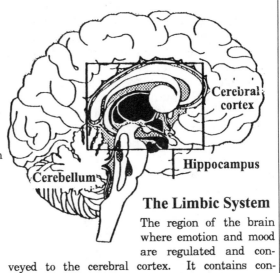

Cerebral cortex

Hippocampus

Cerebellum

The Limbic System

The region of the brain where emotion and mood are regulated and conveyed to the cerebral cortex. It contains concentrations of opiate and dopamine receptors.

Anxiety, panic and grief depletes the brain of amino acids which are the precursors to inhibitory neurotransmitters in the brain. The neurotransmitters are the chemical language of the brain. The amino acids, GABA, glycine, tyrosine, taurine and tryptophan are very important to those who suffer anxiety and fear and should be taken on a daily basis. GABA and glycine are for anxiety. Tyrosine is for depression. Taurine is for the skeletal muscle and central nervous system. Tryptophan is for sleep. Until tryptophan is available, melatonin will be helpful for restful sleep. Amino acids are an extremely important part of the healing process.

Tryptophan Update

In November, 1989, the F.D.A. ordered the amino acid tryptophan removed from the public. As of February, 1994 they still have not released it! Tryptophan was used by millions of people for over 40 years. No significant problems were noted until 1988. Then a rare condition known as E.M.S. (Eosinophilia Myalgia Syndrome) surfaced and was traced to one contaminated batch of tryptophan. The problem occurred in the manufacturing phase in tryptophan made by Showa Denko. Showa Denko, a Japanese firm, corrected the error, but the F.D.A. would not release tryptophan to the millions of adults and children who desperately need it. Tryptophan has been cleared by the C.D.C. (Centers for Disease Control) for release. For many without tryptophan, they would have to turn to toxic, addictive drugs.

The F.D.A. has been given documented studies done with pure pharmaceutical grade tryptophan and the contaminated batch tryptophan. Utilizing the pure tryptophan produced NO problems, but problems existed with the contaminated tryptophan. Tryptophan is safe! This should have proved the point, but the battle rages on.

Indications from the F.D.A. indicate they are considering removing ALL amino acids from the public, and available *only* with a prescription. This means an office visit plus a cost increase of 500% from pharmaceutical industry. Amino acids are the components of proteins. If the F.D.A succeeds with this they might well take away all nutrients.

I took tryptophan for years when it was available. I never saw any problem with my patients nor did I have any myself. If tryptophan is _so unsafe,_ why is it added to every baby formula on the market. If tryptophan becomes a drug, we have lost the battle to Big Brother, God Help Us!

It is important to let your elected representatives in Washington know how you feel. Write, call and visit them. Congress controls the F.D.A., and we can have the freedom to choose natural instead of legalized addictive prescription drugs.

How to Stop "P. A."s
(Panic Attacks)

1. It does not matter if you feel frightened, bewildered, unreal, unsteady. These feelings are nothing more than an exaggeration of the normal bodily reactions to stress.
2. Just because you have these sensations doesn't mean you are very sick. These feelings are just unpleasant and frightening, not dangerous. Nothing worse will happen to you.
3. Let your feelings come. They've been in charge of you. You've been pumping them up and making them more acute. Stop pumping. Don't run away from panic. When you feel the panic mount, take a deep breath and as you breathe out, let go. Keep trying. Stay there almost as if you were floating in space. Don't fight the feeling of panic. Accept it. You can do it.
4. Try to make yourself as comfortable as possible without escaping. If you're on a street, lean against a post or stone wall. If you're at the cosmetic department of the department store, find a quieter counter or corner. If you're in a boutique tell the salesperson you don't feel well and want to sit for a while. Do not jump into your car and go home in fear.
5. Stop adding to your panic with frightening thoughts about what is happening and where it might lead. Don't indulge in self-pity and think, "Why can't I be like all the other, normal people? Why do I have to go through all this?" Just accept what is happening to you. If you do this, what you fear most will not happen.
6. Think about what is really happening to your body at this moment. Do not think, "Something terrible is going to happen. I must get out." Repeat to yourself, "I will not fall, faint, die, or lose control."
7. Now wait and give the fear time to pass. Do not run away. Others have found the strength. You will too.

Notice that as you stop adding the frightening thoughts to your panic, the fear starts to fade away by itself.

8. This is your opportunity to practice. Think of it that way. Even if you feel isolated in space, one of these days you will not feel that way. Sometime soon you will be able to go through the panic and say, "I did it!" Once you say this, you will have gone a long way toward conquering fear. Think about the progress you have already made. You are in the situation!

9. Try to distract yourself from what is going on inside you. Look at your surroundings. See the other people on the street, in the bus. They are with you, not against you.

10. When the panic subsides, let your body go loose, take a deep breath, and go on with your day. Remember, each time you cope with a panic, you reduce your fear.

How to Take a Pill or Capsule

(According to the American Medical Association)

The right way to make the medicine go down depends on whether it is a pill or a capsule.

You won't have to worry about aspirin sticking to the roof of your mouth or vitamins lodging in your throat if you follow this simple procedure.

With a full glass of water at hand, for a tablet, place the pill on your tongue, tilt your head back, and take a swallow of water.

The procedure is similar for a capsule, except that you should tilt your head or upper body *forward*. Since capsules are lighter than water, they will float to the back of your mouth and go down smoothly.

Hyperventilation

An insidious condition, gradually developing over a period of years, in which the victim unconsciously over-breathes, releasing too much carbon dioxide from his body. It is a remarkably prevalent disorder, affecting to some extent a fifth of all adults. And it tends to be unnerving, since hyperventilation can be a marvelous mimic of such diverse disorders as stroke, epilepsy, multiple sclerosis and heart disease. It is by far the most common cause of dizziness, breathlessness, and numbness around the lips or in the limbs in younger people. It can also produce nausea, tremulousness, cold hands and feet, palpitations, and chest pain—the latter often misdiagnosed as a coronary initially when the pain is accompanied by alarming changes in the electrocardiogram.

Most chronic hyperventilators are unaware of their overbreathing. A physician is seldom able to detect this abnormal breathing pattern unless he provokes its characteristic symptoms by having the patient deliberately hyperventilate.

How are hyperventilators treated? A simple explanation of the disorder (along with the strong reassurance that it does not represent some life-threatening disease of the heart, lungs, or brain) and instructions on how to breathe properly usually work wonders. Also, careful instruction in such preventive maneuvers as prolonged breath-holding, or rebreathing carbon dioxide-rich expired air through a paper bag.

If these techniques do not prevent further attacks, another approach can be tried—biofeedback and self hypnosis training. I hyperventilated at one time during my phobic year and found this to be the most effective.

Supplements Available to Consumers Which Could Assist in Fear and Stress Reduction

GABA. Gamma-aminobutyric acid is an amino acid complex which, when taken with niacinamide and inositol, calms anxiety and stress reactions.

L-tyrosine. Recent clinical findings which show that the natural amino acid L-tyrosine is helpful in overcoming depression, improving memory, and increasing mental alertness have stimulated interest in the nutritional role of this dietary factor. Of particular interest is the research linking L-tyrosine deficiency to the development of depression in some oral contraceptive users.

The body needs L-tyrosine to build many complex structural proteins and enzymes, but the recent clinical research has centered on the simpler compounds used by the body to transmit nerve impulses and to determine one's mental mood and alertness. These compounds are called neurotransmitters, and they are readily formed in the body by minor alteration of the L-tyrosine molecule. It is very likely that deficiencies of L-tyrosine can impair the body's ability to produce the proper balance of these neurotransmitters.

In assessing the dietary quantity of L-tyrosine, the L-phenylalanine content of the diet should also be determined, as the body can make L-tyrosine out of "left over" L-phenylalanine. Dietary L-tyrosine can spare the body of some (but not all) of its L-phenylalanine need. The best food sources of L-tyrosine are meats, eggs, and dairy products. Clinical researchers prefer to use L-tyrosine supplements rather than rely on whole foods because it is difficult to obtain such amounts in normal diets.

L-tyrosine (or its precursor, L-phenylalanine) is used by the body to produce several compounds which are important to nerve transmission. The adrenal medulla and nerve cells can quickly produce these compounds from L-tyrosine. The conversions proceed as follows:

L-tyrosine ➜ dopa ➜ dopamine
➜ norepinephrine ➜ epinephrine

Two of these compounds—epinephrine and norepinephrine—have wide-ranging activities which affect brain and nerve cells. Both compounds are produced in nerve cells, as well as in the adrenal medulla where they can be stored. A third compound produced from L-tyrosine—dopamine—affects nerve tracts in the brain, in addition to its role in the production of the other two.

These compounds are called "neurotransmitters" because they control the basic process of impulse transmission between nerve cells. Epinephrine is released at sympathetic nerve (fight-or-flight response) endings, and thus affects the immediate postsynaptic cells. Dopamine transmission appears to be defective in Parkinson's disease.

These neurotransmitters are responsible for an elevated and positive mood, alertness, and ambition. Medical researchers in the past have relied on increasing the brain and nerve levels of norepinephrine by using drugs, such as phenylpropanolamine and amphetamines, which cause the release of norepinephrine, block its return to storage, or slow the destruction of L-tyrosine. However, such artificial manipulation often leads to depletion of the neurotransmitter and the aggravation of the original problem. The natural solution is to normalize brain and nerve levels of norepinephrine by providing adequate levels of dietary L-tyrosine.

Clinical studies have shown that L-tyrosine controls medication-resistant depression. Two studies published in 1980 are of interest. The first was published in the *American Journal of Psychiatry* by Dr. Alan J. Gelenberg of the Department of Psychiatry at Harvard Medical School. Dr. Gelenberg discussed the role of L-tyrosine in controlling anxiety and depression. He postulated that a lack of available L-tyrosine results in a deficiency of the hormone norepinephrine at a specific brain location, which, in turn, relates to mood problems such as depression.

Dr. Gelenberg treated patients having long-standing depression not responding to standard therapy by administering dietary supplements of L-tyrosine. Within two weeks of daily intakes of 100 milligrams per day of an L-tyrosine supplement, tremendous improvement was noted. Patients were able to discontinue or reduce amphetamines to minimal levels in a matter of weeks.

The second study was published in *Lancet* by Dr. I. Goldberg. Allergy sufferers have also responded well to L-tyrosine supplementation, as well as those on weight-loss programs. Durk Pearson reports that L-tyrosine supplementation is a preferred way to control appetite, rather than phenylpropanolamine or amphetamine administration which causes norepinephrine release only.

Tryptophan. An essential amino acid, tryptophan is necessary to maintain the body in protein balance. When food protein deficient in or lacking tryptophan is fed to the growing or mature individual, such food fails to replace worn-out materials which are lost by the body during the organic activities of its cells, tissues, and organs. The amino acid tryptophan is used up in the vital activities of the body, and it must be replaced to prevent atrophy of the body's structures.

Tryptophan is needed in the diet in order for the body to produce niacin, a B complex vitamin. Niacin deficiency can produce pellagra, a syndrome involving the gastrointestinal tract, the skin, and the nervous system. Tryptophan is vital during pregnancy. In an experiment, healthy pregnant rats were given a diet sufficient in everything but tryptophan. Not one of the animals on the deficient diet produced a litter of young, while other healthy pregnant rats fed tryptophan did.

Tryptophan is one of the few substances capable of passing the blood-brain barrier. It has a variety of important roles in mental activity. Serotonin is a neurotransmitter, one of the chemicals in the brain which helps control moods. To have enough serotonin, you need ample tryptophan, which is essential in its formation. To have enough tryptophan, you need enough B-6, without which tryptophan cannot be formed. Many hyperactive children have low serotonin, tryptophan, and B-6 levels. It appears that tryptophan raises the low levels of blood serotonin. Studies done at the North-Nassau Mental Health Center in Manhasset, New York, demonstrate that sufferers of obsessive-compulsive behavior showed signs of improvement following treatment with tryptophan.

Doctors in England found that women who became depressed during the week after they gave birth had low levels of tryptophan, and those with the severest depression had the lowest tryptophan levels. Studies also show that pre-menstrual and post-menopausal females with depression have a tryptophan metabolism disturbance. Further research indicates that tryptophan is superior to drugs in treating depression. Two groups of depressed patients were treated, one with tryptophan and the other with an antidepressant drug called imipramine. Both groups showed significant improvements but tryptophan had fewer side effects. It has also been shown that psychotics and schizophrenics have low blood levels of tryptophan. The solution to these problems is logically linked with dietary supplementation of tryptophan.

Tryptophan has been proved to be valuable in the treatment of sleep disorders. A study at the Maryland Psychiatric Research Center shows that women with the problem of sleep onset latency exhibit a significant improvement when treated with tryptophan. Tryptophan has been reported to significantly reduce sleep latency in insomniacs without altering sleep stages, and to significantly increase total sleep time in insomniac groups. The Sleep Laboratory at Boston State Hospital also confirms the usefulness of this substance in reducing the amount of time it takes to fall asleep and increasing the time spent sleeping.

Parkinson's disease is characterized by tremors. A French study has shown that tryptophan works well in controlling tremors. Twenty people whose severe trembling could not be relieved by L-dopa or other drugs were given 10 grams of tryptophan by mouth daily. In eleven patients, the tremors were satisfactorily controlled.

Siberian Ginseng. Chronic stress results in chronic chemical imbalances in the body. Siberian ginseng, the "adaptogenic herb," increases the body's resistance to life's pressure and strain. Nota W. Nichols, M.D. (Doctor of Herbal Medicine and a medical researcher), states that Siberian ginseng is the state-of-the-art in herbal therapeutics. Research shows that Siberian ginseng has been used for over 5,000 years in China, Korea, and India.

Niacinamide assists in producing tryptophan which is known as the natural relaxant. It is part of the B complex group known as the "stress fighters."

Magnesium Ortate is a mineral found in relatively high amounts in the body. Magnesium is involved in many essential metabolic processes; it helps in the absorption and metabolism of other minerals such as calcium, phosphorus, sodium, and potassium. It also assists in the utilization of the B complex and vitamins C and E. Magnesium is necessary for proper functioning of the nerves, muscles, and neuromuscular contractions. It acts as a relaxant.

Valerian Root is an herb that helps provide prompt overall calming of the nerves and restores a sense of control and balance.

DLPA—DL-phenylalanine—is a nutritional amino acid. Dr. Arnold Fox, in his book *DLPA to End Chronic Pain and Depression*, says that it helps the body to heal itself. DLPA is also a safe anti-depressant and has no side effects. Fox says, "The 10 million people seriously disabled by depression can join the 70 million people who are crippled by chronic pain and arthritis in looking to DLPA for relief."

Glutamine, the amino acid, has been shown to be important in treating alcoholism, sustaining mental ability, and in the treatment of mental-emotional illness.

This nutrient is associated with brain metabolism. While it is nutritionally nonessential for the body as a whole, it is an unique substance in that it can be used—in addition to glucose—as a fuel by brain cells in their very active metabolism. The protective barrier of the brain, the "blood-brain barrier" is very selective and few substances pass through it. Glutamic acid itself does not readily pass through. The amide of glutamic acid, glutamine, does cross the blood-brain barrier. After it gets to the brain, it is transformed into glutamic acid and then used as fuel.

Glutamine protects microorganisms from alcohol poisoning. Given to rats, it gets to the brain and protects the cells so that the rats decrease their voluntary alcohol consumption. Through research at the Pain & Stress Center in San Antonio, alcoholic patients given glutamine voluntarily stopped drinking and stopped having cravings for alcohol for at least two years following the administration of glutamine.

A researcher who gave glutamic acid to schizophrenic patients had limited success in that they improved but only for a few days. These results do suggest that there may be some link between schizophrenic behavior and a lapse in brain metabolism.

Glutamine has been given by mouth to treat toricollis, a condition of contracted cervical muscles also known as wry neck.

Supplements of glutamic acid and glutamine have brought behavior improvement in elderly patients with psychiatric illness. Dr. Carlton Fredericks, in his book *Psycho-Nutrition*, states that he has seen rises of I.Q.'s of children given glutamic acid. He says that although responses differ in degree, occasionally 9 or 10 grams of glutamic acid daily will produce impressive improvements in the ability to learn, to retain, and to recall.

Phobia Dictionary

*Following is a non-inclusive list of phobias
and the fears they represent.*

ACROPHOBIA - heights
AEROPHOBIA - high objects,
  heights or flying
AGORAPHOBIA - open places
AICHMOPHOBIA - knives
AILUROPHOBIA - cats
ALGOPHOBIA - pain
ANDROPHOBIA - men
ANEMOPHOBIA - winds
AGYROPHOBIA - crossing
  streets
ACHLUOPHOBIA - darkness
ANTLOPHOBIA - floods
ASTRAPHOBIA - lightning
ASTHENOPHOBIA - weakness
ARACHNOPHOBIA - spiders
BACCILOPHOBIA - microbes
BACTERIOPHOBIA - bacteria
BATHOPHOBIA - depth
BATOPHOBIA - high buildings
BELONEPHOBIA - pins
  and needles
BROMIDROSIPHOBIA - body
  odor
CANCERPHOBIA - cancer
CLAUSTROPHOBIA - con-
  finement
COPROSTASOPHOBIA - con-
  stipation
CLINOPHOBIA - beds
CYNOPHOBIA - dogs
CARDIOPHOBIA - heart
  disease
DECIDOPHOBIA - making
  decisions
DOMATOPHOBIA - being
  confined in a house
DEMONOPHOBIA - demons

DENTAL PHOBIA - dentists
DIABETOPHOBIA - Diabetes
DIKEPHOBIA - police
DERMATOPHATHOPHOBIA
  - skin disease
ENTOMOPHOBIA - insects
EPISTEMOPHOBIA - school
EREMOPHOBIA - being alone
ELECTROPHOBIA - electricity
EROTOPHOBIA - sex
EMETOPHOBIA - vomiting
EQUINOPHOBIA - horses
ERGOPHOBIA - work
GALEOPHOBIA - cats
GAMOPHOBIA - marriage
GEPHYROPHOBIA - crossing
  bridges
GERONTOPHOBIA - old age
GYMNOPHOBIA - nudity
GYNEPHOBIA - women
HAGIOPHOBIA - church
HEMAPHOBIA - blood
HYDROPHOBIA - water
HOMICHLOPHOBIA - fog
HIPPOPHOBIA - horses
HYPEGIAPHOBIA - responsi-
  bility
HORMEPHOBIA - shock
HYPNOPHOBIA - sleep
HODOPHOBIA - traveling
IATROPHOBIA - doctors
KERAUNOPHOBIA - thunder
KAKORRAPHIAPHOBIA -
  failure
KATAGELOPHOBIA - ridicule
LALOPHOBIA - speaking
  in public
LYSSOPHOBIA - insanity

MONOPHOBIA - one thing
MYSOPHOBIA - germs or contamination and dirt
MASTIGOPHOBIA - beating
MENINGITOPHOBIA - meningitis
MUSOPHOBIA - mice
NECROPHOBIA - dead bodies
NEPHOPHOBIA - clouds
NUCLEOMITIPHOBIA - nuclear bombs
NYCTOPHOBIA - night
OCHLOPHOBIA - crowds
OMBROPHOBIA - rain
OPTOPHOBIA - opening one's eyes
ORNITHOPHOBIA - birds
OPHIDIOPHOBIA, OPHIO-PHOBIA - snakes
PANTOPHOBIA - fears
PATHOPHOBIA - disease
PECCATOPHOBIA - sinning
PELADOPHOBIA - baldness
PHOBOPHOBIA - one's own fears
PSYCHROPHOBIA - cold
PYROPHOBIA - fire
PHARMACOPHOBIA - drugs
PATRIOPHOBIA - negative traits in parents
PENIAPHOBIA - poverty
POINEPHOBIA - punishment
POLISOPHOBIA - cities

PNIGOPHOBIA or PNIGERO-PHOBIA - smothering
PHAGOPHOBIA - swallowing
PHASMOPHOBIA - ghosts
PYROPHOBIA - fires
SYPHILOPHOBIA - syphilis
SPERMOPHOBIA or SPERMATOPHOBIA - germs
SELACHOPHOBIA - sharks
SELAPHOBIA - light flashes
SCIOPHOBIA - shadows
TAPHEPHOBIA - being buried alive
THALASSOPHOBIA - the ocean
THANATOPHOBIA - death
TOPOPHOBIA - performing (stage fright)
TROPOPHOBIA - moving or making change
TRICHOPHOBIA - hair
TOCOPHOBIA - childbirth
THEOPHOBIA - God
TREMOPHOBIA - trembling
TRICHNIOPHOBIA - trichinosis
TRISKAIDEKAPHOBIA - number thirteen
TUBERCULOPHOBIA - tuberculosis
VERBOPHOBIA - words
XENOPHOBIA - strangers
ZOOPHOBIA - animals

Resources

A wide range of reference books is listed to assist those who wish to educate themselves further. You will notice that each presents a totally different approach to treatment of anxiety, fear, and phobias. Most physicians and researchers disagree with each other's philosophy. I feel the material presented in this text, *The Anxiety Epidemic*, will give the reader a new approach, insight, and information which has not been previously published.

I wish to acknowledge here that Dr. Kenneth Pelletier's book *Mind as Healer, Mind as Slayer* opened many avenues of understanding for me in the area of psychosomatic medicine. Dr. Pelletier introduced in 1977 the mental physical symptom syndrome in such a way that one's understanding took on a new dimension.

Adams, Ruth and Frank Murray. *Mega Vitamin Therapy.* Larchmont Books.

Austin, Phylis, et al. *Food Allergies Made Simple.* New Lifestyle Books.

Bland, Jeffrey, Ph.D. Ed, *Medical Applications of Clinical Nutrition.* Keats Publishing.

Blum, Kenneth, Ph.D. *Handbook of Abusable Drugs.* Gardner Press.

Bresler, David, Ph.D. with Richard Trubo. *Free Yourself From Pain.* Simon and Schuster.

Chaitow, Leon, D.O. *Thorsons Guide to Amino Acids.* Thorsons Publishing.

Cousins, Norman. *The Healing Heart.* Avon Books.

Gelb, Harold, D.M.D. *Killing Pain Without a Prescription.* Harper & Row.

Green, Bernard, Ph.D. *Goodbye Blue: Breaking The Tranquilizer Habit The Natural Way.* McGraw Hill.

Hay, Louise L. *Overcoming Fears* cassette. Hay House Audio.

Hoffer, Abram, M.D. Ph.D. and Morton Walker, D.P.M. *Orthomolecular Nutrition.* Keats / Pivot.

Lesser, Michael, M.D. *Nutrition and Vitamin Therapy.* Bantam Books.

Murphy, Joseph, Ph.D. *The Power of Your Subconscious Mind.* Prentice-Hall.

Pelletier, Kenneth R. *Mind as Healer, Mind as Slayer.* Dell Publishing Co., Inc.

Rapp, Doris J., M.D. *Allergies & Your Family.* Practical Allergy Research Foundation.

Rapp, Doris J. M.D. *Recognize and Manage Your Allergies.* Practical Allergy Research Foundation.

Rapp, Doris J., M.D. *Is This Your Child?* William Morrow and Co., Inc.

Ricketts, Max with Edwin Bien. *The Great Anxiety Escape.* Matulungin Publishing.

Sahley, Billie J., Ph.D. *Anxiety* cassette. Pain & Stress Therapy Center Publications.

Sahley, Billie J., Ph.D. *Anxiety / Panic Attacks,* Pain & Stress Therapy Center Publications.

Sahley, Billie J., Ph.D. and Katherine M. Birkner, C.R.N.A., Ph.D. *Breaking Your Addiction Habit.* Pain & Stress Therapy Center Publications.

Sahley, Billie J., Ph.D. *Chronic Emotional Fatigue.* Pain & Stress Therapy Center Publications.

Sahley, Billie J., Ph.D. and Katherine M. Birkner C.R.N.A., Ph.D., *Therapeutic Use of Amino Acids* cassette. Pain & Stress Therapy Publications.

Seigal, Bernie, M.D. *Love, Medicine and Miracles.* Harper & Row.

Seigal, Bernie, M.D. "Prescription For Living" Series of Cassettes. Hay House Audio.

Slagle, Priscilla. *The Way Up From Down.* St. Martin's Publishing.

Wade, Carleson. *Vitamins, Minerals, and Other Supplements.* Keats / Pivot.

Weeks, Clare, M.D. *More Help For Your Nerves.* Bantam Books.

Wolfe, J. *The Practice of Behavior Therapy.* Permagon Press.

Wood, John T. *What Are You Afraid Of?* Prentice-Hall.

Wright, Jonathon, M.D. *Dr. Wright's Book of Nutritional Therapy.* Rodale Press.

X
UPDATE

Eight years have passed since I wrote the first edition of *The Anxiety Epidemic*. It has been a time of discovery and learning, a time of reinforcement that prescription drugs are not the answer to anxiety, panic or fear and they never will be! I thank God for the courage to keep fighting and the strength to keep searching for natural alternatives to help those who walk the lonely path as I did.

As for all of those patients whose symptoms I described on previous pages. They are all healed and live in peace. I'm especially happy for Sister Karen, she is now Mother Superior in a very large convent. She has not experienced any more of the old problems. But in times of prolonged stress, she keeps her neurotransmitter formula handy. Sister Karen had a major deficiency of amino acids and magnesium. She was as depleted as I was after my traumatic years.

A therapist's life is always busy. Although I enjoy my work, it is very demanding. I keep myself on an amino acid and nutrient regime, take time for meditation, and never, ever forget my magnesium. If I had known what a magnesium deficiency can cause, I could have avoided so much suffering.

Over the past years I have seen a multitude of patients from all walks of life with anxiety, panic, fear and phobias. They all feel their symptoms are unique, and no one else could suffer as much as they have. Little do they know. Most of them had given in to what they thought would be freedom, prescription drugs. What they found out was, they were living in a chemical straight jacket!

The pharmaceutical industry, the world's most profitable business, promises new life. No fear and anxiety if you will just take their pills. Their power and influence is awesome. They thrive on illness and weakness, not health and well being.

In January, 1993 the truth came out. *Consumer Reports* magazine, did an independent study of all of the F.D.A. approved antidepressants and tranquilizers. What did this study reveal? The drugs didn't work. They are not the answer to stress induced pain, anxiety, depression, grief or fear. One of the biggest challenges you will face is constantly being offered prescription drugs by well meaning physicians who think they are helping you.

When I think about what would have happened to me and how my life would have turned out if I had not said no. I know someone was watching over me.

With the Lord's help, all of those patients who have come in searching for answers are now healed and live in peace. All of the drugs in the world won't put a face on the fear or resolve anxiety, your life becomes an endless search for an answer. But the right amino acids and nutrient program, finding a therapist with empathic understanding, will give you your keys to a safe, long term recovery.

PANIC ATTACK OR ALLERGIC REACTION?

Allergies don't just cause sniffles and itchy eyes. Few physicians and even fewer patients are aware that ordinary allergies, food, airborne or chemical sensitivities can cause psychological reactions. Symptoms range from mood swings and depression to full-blown panic attacks.

Since panic attacks are no longer uncommon, most physicians are likely to suspect a psychological problem when the culprit could be a food allergy or other sensitivity that won't show up in standard allergy tests. There were many times during my personal episode I would experience what I thought was a panic attack . . .rapid heart beat, shortness of breath, irritability, and tension. These sensations continued even after I was on a good orthomolecular program, and my grief and depression resolved for the most part. Determined to stop all of the old feelings, I began to research what could possibly cause the physical symptoms I was experiencing. I focused on the accelerated heartbeat in relation to allergic reactions because I knew I got a sick headache from certain odors. The formaldehyde fumes from a new carpet in my home were literally driving me crazy every night. I was experiencing chemical pain.

Then, as I went through the symptoms of food allergy I realized what I thought was a panic attack was in fact, an allergic reaction to milk. I always had digestive problems with milk, so did my mother. At that time I thought the best thing I could eat was yogurt. So I did everyday I could. Because of my reactions I knew it had to be a severe allergy. So I stopped all dairy products. Forty-eight hours later the symptoms stopped. The tendency to develop food allergies is increased if the intestinal lining has been damaged for any reason. One example of this is a person who has regular diarrhea or irritable bowel syndrome. The intestinal wall becomes porous, then loses some of its normal protective lining or immune barriers.

Oddly enough, the foods you crave the most are the ones you could have a food allergy to. If you think this could be one of your problems with one or more foods, there are tests available. It only requires one blood draw for accurate results. A quick way to check, when you are having the symptoms, is to take an *Alka Seltzer Gold.* It has the ability to neutralize a food reaction and the symptoms will stop in minutes. Make sure you use only the *Alka Selzer Gold.*

Doris Rapp, M.D. has done extensive research in this area and has published several books. Dr. Rapp's research established there are thousand of children in this country who are given Ritalin, a very powerful drug for hyperactivity, when in fact, their problem is food, airborne or chemical allergies. Both food and chemical sensitivities can and do alter a person's ability to learn and concentrate.

I've had several hundred patients come to the Pain & Stress Center who described these symptoms in detail. Over half of them had seen a physician, you guessed it, they were given Xanax or Ritalin for food and airborne allergies. They were tested and the foods withdrawn from their diets for at least 30 days. The next step was a food rotation diet.

Allergy sufferers respond to a balanced hypoallergenic supplement program. The amino acid, tyrosine, is very helpful. It helps to fortify the immune system especially because one breakdown product of tyrosine is epinephrine. Tyrosine is used by the environmental medicine doctors to treat acute episodes of allergic reactions. If you suspect this could be one of your problems, keep a food diary and note down how you feel after you eat certain foods. An excellent resource is *Allergies & Your Family* by Doris Rapp, M.D.

For those who have airborne allergies, you need at least 5000 mg of Ester C daily. Ester C has a pH of 7.0 which means its as neutral as distilled water. So you will not experience any adverse side effects from Ester C that you might have with regular Vitamin C. Ester C is safe for children and infants.

In this update I have tried to bring you forward from 1986 to the present. As my own search began for answers to my pain and suffering, it ended with a new direction in my life. I have fulfilled my impossible dream because I am living it. I won't deny that there haven't been times when the past has tried to sneak in and pull me back. It has. I don't have any anxiety or panic attacks, but I do find myself wondering what my life would have been like if I had not been burned at 14 months and lost my father at age 6. I had a very abusive stepfather who constantly rejected me, and mistreated my mother. I have worked very hard to deal with it and let it go, and I have for the most part. But still I feel the grief, especially when I think what it might have been like to call someone Dad. Then I return to the present, hearing the words, "Peace be with you, now go and do what I have chosen."

Dominus vobiscum.

GABA, THE BRAIN AND BEHAVIOR

The study of GABA and other amino acids, how they affect the brain and behavior is making a significant contribution to the understanding of disease in man. Disease is now being found to arise from causes within the person such as nutrient imbalances and the body's reaction to stress as well as environmental changes of the brain's chemistry. These changes, can and do cause a difference in perception.

The various functions of amino acids are the most important and diverse healers within the body. A new age of medicine has emerged and has substantial evidence that nutrient deficiencies can and do influence mind, mood, memory and behavior. Amino acid requirements in the body and brain are vastly increased by disease and inborn metabolic errors. Anytime a person is under prolonged periods of stress, anxiety, depression or grief, they require more amino acids, some more than others. The reason for the different requirements is biochemical individuality.

Every individual has a distinct chemical composition. The brain, glands and bones are distinct for each individual, not only in anatomy, but also in chemical composition. This does not mean that chemical compositions are fixed throughout life or that they are not influenced by nutrition. Nutrition and amino acid deficiencies effect every tissue in the body. The kidneys stop functioning, the stomach stops digesting, the adrenals stop secreting, and other organs follow suit.

GABA (Gamma Amino Butyric Acid), an inhibitory transmitter, is found throughout the central nervous system (CNS). In view of our growing knowledge, regarding the regulation of physiology of the CNS, GABA is assuming an ever-enlarging role as a major influence on drugs, in many cases replacing them. The most valid scientific research published on GABA relate to how it effects anxiety / stress in the brain.

Let's examine a step-by-step process of what happens in the brain to begin the cycle of stress and anxiety, and how GABA works in your brain. Panic, anxiety or stress related messages begin to release numerous signals, and concurrently, a physiological response begins to take place..the fight or flight syndrome; you feel as though everything inside of you is going off at once. You have NO control.

The unceasing alert signals from the limbic system eventually overwhelms the cortex (the decision making part of the brain) and the ability of the cortex and the rest of the stress network becomes exhausted. The balance between the limbic system, and in fact, the rest of the brain to communicate in an orderly manner depends critically on inhibition. GABA inhibits the cells from firing, diminishing the anxiety related messages from reaching the cortex.

What GABA does is fill certain receptor sites in the brain; this slows down or blocks the excitatory levels of the brain cells that are about to receive the incoming information. When the message is received by the cortex, it does not overwhelm you with anxiety, panic or pain. You are able to maintain control and remain calm. But if you are under prolonged stress or anxiety, your brain uses up all the available GABA; this then allows anxiety, fear, panic, and pain to hit you from every direction. Your ability to reason is diminished, the effects can now include a full blown anxiety or panic attack, excessive sweating, trembling, muscle tension, weakness, loss of control, disorientation, difficulty in breathing, constant fear, headaches, diarrhea, depression, unsteady legs, the list is endless.

Research done at The Pain & Stress Therapy Center in San Antonio with patients suffering from all types of stress, pain, muscle spasms or anxiety / panic attacks has shown pure GABA 750 mg can mimic the tranquilizing effects of Valium, Librium, or a multitude of other tranquilizers, but *without* the possibility of addiction or fear of being sedated. GABA fills the receptor in the brain and feeds the brain what should be there.   Pure GABA dissolves in water; it is tasteless, odorless, and the calming results usually occur within 7 minutes.

Tranquilizers are only a temporary coating, but a very dangerous one.   We have seen many patients who are on Xanax when they come in with anxiety. They have been told it is not addicting....it is! Xanax will not stop anxiety or panic nor can it feed the brain the nutrients it needs. *THERE IS NO SUCH THING AS A TRANQUILIZER DEFICIENCY*--- nutrient deficiencies do change behavior.   Human behavior involves the functioning of the whole nervous system, and the nervous system requires amino acids. GABA is vital for energy and the smooth running of the brain functions.

GABA, itself, is an inhibiting neurotransmitter and is known to be a calming agent in the brain. B6 (pyridoxine) is GABA's most important partner. We have successfully used GABA with patients to ease anxiety, muscle pain / spasms, and nervous stomachs.   The GABA we use is freeform, not combined with anything else.   There is a GABA with niacinamide and inositol on the market, but let me caution you---do not megadose, as you will have side effects.   It is best when you combine GABA with other amino acids that control your stress and anxiety.   Over the past years, we have done extensive research using amino acids in many areas of health, but especially anxiety, stress, depression and pain.   The public is now taking a serious interest in their health. This interest will bring GABA and other amino acids to the forefront of health care.

MAGNESIUM, THE MIRACLE MINERAL

Over the past several years the focus has been calcium for the prevention and treatment of osteoporosis, to lower high blood pressure and to keep muscles in the body operating properly. Few people if any know that magnesium is needed for the same reason plus many more.

In the process of trying to get sufficient amounts of calcium, most everyone pays little attention to their intake of magnesium.

Like calcium, magnesium also helps assure that you have strong bones and teeth, lowers high blood pressure and maintains muscle health. WHILE CALCIUM IS NEEDED FOR MUSCLE CONTRACTION, MAGNESIUM IS REQUIRED FOR MUSCLE RELAXATION. Some recent research shows that magnesium is needed in a balance of 2 parts: 1 part calcium.

According to Sherry Rogers, M.D., conditions that may be associated with magnesium deficiency include: gastrointestinal disorders such as malabsorption syndromes due to sprue, bowel resection, prolonged diarrhea, alcoholic cirrhosis, and pancreatitis. Other conditions associated with magnesium deficiency are anxiety and panic attacks, osteoarthritis, depression, hyperactivity, eclampsia, premenstrual syndrome, hyperthyroidism, insomnia, cardiovascular disease, excessive perspiration, and body odor. Diuretic therapy, excessive lactation, renal disease and endocrine disorders also have magnesium deficiency reports.

Many people have spastic conditions which clearly are caused by a deficiency of magnesium. This includes asthma, migraine, colitis, angina, chronic back pain, muscle spasms, arrythmias, vasculitis, hypertension, eye twitches, cystitis, tremors, seizures, Raynaud's disease, infertility and nystagmus. But vertigo (dizziness), psychosis, confusion, eclampsia, diabetes, phlebitis, exhaustion, T.I.A.'s (transient spasms of arteries in head), refractoriness to potassium therapy and insulin can also be due to magnesium deficiency.

All patients with anxiety and panic attacks at the Pain & Stress Therapy Center are put on magnesium. Usually Slow-Mag is used, and they improve within 48 hours. Slow-Mag is a time released magnesium. Magnesium chloride is efficiently absorbed in the alkaline area of the small intestine. For those taking magnesium supplements, there should not be a problem with adverse reaction unless you have kidney disease. The kidneys compensate for an excess uptake by increasing urinary excretion of magnesium.

I have found that my body requires six Slow-Mag per day, spaced throughout the day. The most common side effect from magnesium supplementation is loose stools or diarrhea. This is welcome relief for anyone who has suffered from chronic constipation. You must be patient and find your body's optimal dose. In addition, magnesium solution, 1 teaspoon once or twice per day provides additional magnesium. Results with maximum improvement have been noted.

Most people short change themselves in magnesium along with other critically needed nutrients. Although the R.D.A. for magnesium is 400 mg, the typical American diet supplies between 200-300 mg daily.

Many patients ask what test they could run to find out just how deficient they are. Blood tests like C.B.C. (complete blood count) or R.B.C. (red blood cell) magnesium and the plasma magnesium are practically useless. In most people it comes back normal yet the person exhibits magnesium deficiency signs and symptoms. These tests miss about 80% of the people that are deficient in magnesium.

Dr. Jon Pangborn suggests that if specific amino acids are low in a 24 hour urine amino acid analysis, you can be pretty sure that you have a magnesium deficiency. Magnesium levels can also be determined with collection of a 24 hour urine. Then load challenges of magnesium are given and another 24 hour urine is collected for analysis of magnesium uptake and excretion. So urine, not blood will be the true test of what the body needs.

One of the most common symptoms of magnesium deficient patients are those with constant, chronic back and neck pain. Since I began using it for an old auto accident whiplash, I have felt like my old self. For those who are in a great deal of pain, we use I.V. magnesium so the therapists can work on them without discomfort. Magnesium deficiency is one of the causes of protracted muscle spasms, stiff and sore muscles upon awakening, and anxiety.

And magnesium deficiency causes the body to release more histamine. Histamine is released whenever you react to an allergen which triggers an allergic reaction. This can be environmental, chemical or food. A reaction to a food can trigger symptoms that mimic an anxiety attack. So be aware of your body and ask if you are really having an anxiety attack.

Life is said to begin at 40, but I'm afraid the same cannot be said of bone mass. At the age of 35, after reaching its peak, bone mass starts to decline due to an imbalance of the modeling process and bones start to lose both their mineral and their gelatinous matrix. Women in menopause or change of life begin a bone crisis. At this time a rapid decrease in bone mass occurs. Thus, we see women sustaining more fractures than those taking a regular supplement program that includes enough magnesium.

In summary, remember several major points. As with many minerals, the average diet is deficient in magnesium. The diet only provides 40% of the R.D.A. It is estimated by Dr. Mildred Seelig, a nationally recognized magnesium specialist, that over 80% of the population is low. Do you think you should consider adding magnesium to your supplement program? Considering all of the available research done--- you should certainly reevaluate your current health status.

TAURINE

Taurine is a naturally occurring amino acid that is highly concentrated in animal and fish proteins, especially organ meats. It is manufactured in the body from methionine or cysteine in the liver when B6 is present. Taurine is found in appreciable amounts in excitable tissue as the heart, skeletal muscle, eye, and the central nervous system including the brain. Taurine is the most plentiful amino acid in the developing brain and the second most abundant in the brain after glutamic acid. It is no wonder that disturbances in taurine metabolism are seen in problems as diverse as heart disease and epilepsy.

Taurine protects and stabilizes the brain's fragile membranes and acts as a neurotransmitter. It seems to be closely related in its structure and metabolism to other neurotransmitters such as glycine and GABA. Taurine, like GABA, is inhibitory. Taurine, or a modified taurine, may someday supersede synthetic tranquilizers.

Women require more taurine than men since estradiol is found to inhibit its synthesis in the liver.

Some studies found significantly decreased levels of taurine in depressed patients. This has been confirmed with amino acid analysis.

Taurine has a potent anticonvulsant action. Most studies find taurine is diminished in epileptic and seizure patients. Taurine intakes between 200 and 1500 mg per day have been helpful in epileptic seizures. However, higher does of taurine may be required. Taurine has been found to assist people with tics or other spastic conditions.

Taurine improves fat metabolism in the liver, seems to play a role with cholesterol and in the formation of gall stones. Taurine helps to conserve potassium and calcium in the heart muscle, thereby helping the heart to function better. As with most nutrients, the body's need for taurine increases whenever an individual is under stress.

GLYCINE

Glycine is the simplest nonessential amino acid. It resembles glucose (blood sugar) and glycogen (liver starch). Glycine is sweet to taste and can be used as a sweetener. It can mask bitterness and saltiness. Pure glycine dissolves easily in liquids. Glycine is probably the third major inhibitory neurotransmitter of the brain. Glycine readily passes the blood-brain barrier.

Although glycine is not an essential amino acid, it is an essential intermediate in the metabolism of protein, peptides, and bile salts. Glycine, taurine and GABA are the major inhibitory neurotransmitters in the brain and C.N.S. Glycine is a very nontoxic amino acid. Even with doses up to 30 grams glycine has not produced side effects.

Glycine is thought to be involved in behaviors related to convulsions and retinal function. Glycine taken orally will increase the urinary excretion of uric acid. It is possibly a useful adjunct of gout.

Glycine, like taurine, seems to be important in epilepsy and spasticity. In addition, glycine alleviate the toxic effects of substances such as phenol, benzoic acid and lead. Glycine may be used to reduce aggression since glycine can have a sedative effect. In one study, glycine in large doses, ended an acute manic episode within one hour.

MELATONIN

One of the most exciting therapies that has emerged in the last couple of years is clinical use of melatonin.

Melatonin is a potent immune regulator. It is contained in the pineal gland situated in the anterior portion, at the base of the brain. This gland's main hormone is melatonin. Melatonin has been the subject of intense research in Europe and the U.S. The main focus that has attracted so much attention is that melatonin metabolizes in the brain as tryptophan and elevates the serotonin level.

Melatonin regulates our biological clock. It is distinguished as the regulator of the body's circadian rhythm that makes us sleep at night and wake up in the morning. Some researchers consider melatonin a primary regulator of the body's immune system protecting us from all forms of stress. Melatonin's sedative qualities have been shown to decrease anxiety, panic disorders and some migraine headaches.

Serfina Corsello, an orthomolecular doctor, uses melatonin with her patients. Dr. Corsello states she finds melatonin to be one of the most effective interventions in her practice. Patients have reported excellent results for sleep problems. Melatonin is available in 3 mg capsules. One capsule an hour before bed is effective.

B VITAMINS

The B vitamins are synergistic with each other. This simply means that each of the B vitamins works best in the presence of an adequate amount of the others.

As a complex, the B vitamins play a significant role in alleviating depression and in relieving the anxiety and restlessness that often accompanies it, perhaps partially due to the effect of the B vitamins on lactic acid. Certain metabolic processes and exercise produce the formation of lactic acid when there is inadequate B vitamins or oxygen. If you exercise strenuously without gradually building up, lactic acid accumulates in your muscles. But excessive lactic acid can also produce anxiety.

The first clinical effects of inadequate B vitamins are insomnia, mood changes, decrease immune function, impaired drug metabolism and sugar cravings.

VITAMIN B6 (PYRIDOXINE)

Vitamin B6 has a major role in regulating your moods and is often implicated in the cause and treatment of depression.

B6 might better be termed the Enabler vitamin. Vitamin B6 literally controls all the amino acid metabolism and transformations in your body. B6 is required for the proper functioning of over 60 metabolic and enzymatic processes in the body. Without adequate B6, the amino acids are not of much value to you. It also controls amino acid absorption from your gastrointestinal tract. B6 is involved in carbohydrate and fat metabolism as well as the formation of red blood cells and antibodies.

The average American diet tends to be high in protein and fat. This causes an increased requirement of B6. More B6 is depleted by stress, alcohol consumption, tobacco, birth control pills, pregnancy, and medications.

B6 is available in 150 mg timed-release capsules that are released over 9 to 10 hours. Another way to ensure adequate intake of B6 is to use the biological form of B6 or P 5' P (Pyridoxal 5' Phosphate).

In closing, I'd like to quote Pfeiffer's Law from *The Healing Nutrients Within*, "We found that if a drug can be found to do the job of medical healing, a nutrient can be found to do the same job. When we understand how a drug works, we can imitate its action with one of the nutrients."

WARNING: *Rx Drugs Are Drugs*

There are no drugs in pharmacology which cure anxiety, panic phobias, insomnia, depression, asthma, arthritis, diabetes, heart disease, hyperactivity or inflammatory condition, pain or disease.

There are many drugs which treat the symptoms of these disorders. However, many prescription drugs have a significant potential for long term adverse or permanent side effects.

Bibliography

Ashmead, DeWayne. "Lead Toxicity." *Health Express.* October 1983, pp. 16-17.

Benson, Herbert. *The Mind / Body Effect.* New York: Simon and Schuster, 1979.

Bergmann, Kenneth J. "Prozabide: A New GABA-Mimetic Agent in Clinical Use." *Clinical Neuropharmacology.* Vol. 8, No.1, 1985. New York: Raven Press, pp. 13-23.

Bland, Jeffrey, ed. *Medical Applications of Clinical Nutrition.* New Canaan, CN: Keats Publishing, Inc., 1983.

Blum, Kenneth. *Handbook of Abusable Drugs.* New York: Gardner Press, Inc., 1984.

Bond, Michael. *Pain Its Nature, Analysis, and Treatment.* New York: Churchill Livingstone, 1979.

Bourne, Tom. "How to Collect Insurance Claims." *Medical Self-Care.* Fall, 1982, pp. 28-31.

Braestrup, Claus and Nielsen, Mogens. "Neurotransmitters and CNS Disease." *The Lancet.* November, 1982, pp. 1030-1034.

"The Brain" series. Public Broadcasting Service, January, 1985.

Brainard, John B. *Control of Migraines.* New York: W.W. Norton & Co., 1979, pp.1-23.

Braverman, Eric R. and Pfeiffer, Carl C. *The Healing Nutrients Within.* New Canaan, CN: Keats Publishing, Inc., 1987.

Bresler, David E. with Trubo, Richard. *Free Yourself From Pain.* New York: Simon and Schuster, 1979.

Brown, Barbara. *Between Health and Illness.* New York: Bantam Books, 1985.

Brown, C.C. et al. "Effects of L-Tryptophan on Sleep Onset Insomniacs." *Walking and Sleeping.* April, 1979, pp. 101-108.

Callahan, Sheila. "Tension Headaches. What's in a Name?" *Aches and Pains.* October 1980, pp. 14-16.

Challem, Jack Joseph. "Everything You Need to Know About Amino Acids." *Health Quarterly.* Winter, 1982, pp. 13, 60-61.

Cheraskin, E., Ringsdorf, W.M., and Clark, J. W. *Diet and Disease.* New Canaan, CN: Keats Publishing Inc., 1968.

Chweh, A.Y., et al. "Effect of GABA Agonists on Neurotoxicity and Anticonvulsant Activity of Benzodiazepines." *Life Sciences.* Vol. 36, No. 8, 1985, pp. 737-744.

Colby-Morley, Elsa. "Neurotransmitters and Nutrition." *Journal of Orthomolecular Psychiatry.* First Quarter 1983, pp. 38-39.

Cooper, Jack R., et al. . *The Biochemical Basis of Neuropharmacology.* 5th Ed. New York: Oxford Press, 1986.

Cowen, P.J. and Nutt, D.J. "Abstinence Symptoms After Withdrawal of Tranquilizing Drugs: Is There a Common Neurochemical Mechanism?" *The Lancet.* August 14, 1982, pp. 360-362.

Diamond, Seymour and Medina, Joe L. "Headaches." *Clinical Symposia.* Vol. 33, No. 2. Summit, NJ: CIBA Pharmaceutical Co., 1981.

Dietrich, Schneider-Helmert. "Interval Therapy with L-Tryptophan in Severe Chronic Insomniacs." *International Pharmacopsychiatry.* Vol. 16. 1981, pp. 162-173.

Doheny, Kathleen. "Panic Attacks: A Debilitating Disorder for Millions." *Health Express.* June 1983, pp. 60-61.

Donsbach, Kurt W. "Phenylalanine and Depression." *Health Express.* January 1982, p. 40.

------. "Neurotransmitters." *Health Express.* May 1982, p. 58.

Downs, Robert and Van Baak, Alice. "The Amazing Power of Amino Acids, Part I. *Bestways* January 1982, pp. 74-75.
------. "The Amazing Power of Amino Acids, Part II." *Bestways.* February 1982, pp. 56-58.

"Emotions in Pain," *Pain Current Concepts on Pain and Analgesia.* Vol. 5, No. 1, pp 1-2.

Ferguson, Marilyn. *The Aquarian Conspiracy, Personal and Social Transformation in the 1980s.* Los Angeles J.P. Tarcher, Inc., 1980.

Fishman, Scott M. and Sheen, David V. "Anxiety and Panic: Their Cause and Treatment." *Psychology Today.* April, 1985., pp. 26-32.

Fredericks, Carton. *New & Complete Nutrition Handbook.* Canoga Park, CA: Major Books, 1976; Reprint ed., Huntington Beach, CA: International Institute of Natural Health Sciences, Inc., 1977.

------. "Hotline to Health." *Prevention Magazine.* February 1979, p.42.

------. "Hotline to Health." *Prevention Magazine.* March 1979, p. 38.

Garrison, Robert Jr. *Lysine, Tryptophan, and Other Amino Acids.* New Canaan, CN: Keats Publishing, Inc., 1982.

Gelb, Harold. *Killing Pain Without a Prescription.* New York: Harper and Row Publishers, 1980.

Gelenberg, Alan J., et al. "Tyrosine For the Treatment of Depression." *American Journal of Psychiatry.* May 1980, pp. 622-623.

Gottlieb, Bill. "Brain Food." *Prevention Magazine.* September 1979, p. 185.

Graedon, Joe and Ferguson, Tom. "Saving Money on Drugs." *Medical Self-Care.* Fall 1982, pp. 24-25.

Grant, Larry A. "Amino Acids in Action." *Let's Live Magazine.* August 1983, p. 61-64.

Guyton, Arthur C. *Basic Human Neurophysiology.* Third Edition. Philadelphia: W.B. Saunders Company, 1981, pp. 207-217, 223.

Hammond, Edward J. and Wilder, B.J. "Gamma-Vinyl GABA: A New Antiepileptic Drug. *Clinical Neuropharmacology.* Vol. 8, No. 1, 1985, pp. 1-12.

Health Express, "Stress Reaction," June 1983, p. 48.

Hench, P. Kahler. "Myofascial Pain Syndromes." *Myology.* Vol. 5, No. 1. A.H. Robins Pharmaceutical, 1980.

Hersen, Michel, et al. *Progress in Behavior Modification.* Vol. 14. New York: Academic Press, 1983.

Hoffer, Abram and Walker, Morton. *Orthomolecular Nutrition.* New Canaan, CN: Keats Publishing Inc., 1978.

Hospital Medicine, "Clinical Highlights," September 1983.

An Introduction to Integral Medicine. 2 Vols. Pacific Palisades, CA: Center for Integral Medicine, 1978.

Iverson, Leslie L. "Neurotransmitters. " *The Lancet.* October 23, 1982. pp. 914-918.

Kaplan, Harold I, Freedman, Alfred, and Sadock, Benjamin. *Comprehensive Textbook of Psychiatry.* Vol. 3. Baltimore: Williams and Wilkins, 1980.

King, Robert B. "Pain and Tryptophan." *Journal Neurosurgery* 53. July 1980, pp. 44-52.

Kolata, Gina. "Your Hungry Brain." *American Health.* May / June 1983, pp. 45-50.

Kraus, Hans. *Clinical Treatment of Back and Neck Pain.* New York: McGraw-Hill Book Company, 1970.

Lee, William H. "Amazing Amino Acids." New Canaan, CN: Pine Grove Pamphlet Division of Keats Publishing, Inc., 1984.

Lesser, Michael. *Nutrition and Vitamin Therapy.* New York: Bantam Books, 1981.

Long, Ruth Yale. "Foods for Improving Mental Health." *Bestways.* January 1982, pp. 36-37.

Mann, John, et al. "D-Phenylalanine in Endogenous Depression." *American Journal of Psychiatry.* December 1980, pp. 1611-1612.

Mazer, Eileen. "Tryptophan-The Three Way Misery Reliever." *Prevention Magazine.* May 1983, pp. 134-139.

"National Institute of Mental Health." *Medical World News.* January 1985, p. 17, 20.

New Frontiers in Pain control: Alternatives to Drugs and Surgery. Pacific Palisades, CA: Center for Integral Medicine, 1978.

Pearson, Durk and Shaw, Sandy. *Life Extension.* New York: Warner Books, Inc., 1982.

Pelletier, Kenneth R. *Mind as Healer, Mind as Slayer.* New York: Dell Publishing Co., Inc., 1977.

------. "Mental Stress-Physical Illness." *Psychology Today* Cassettes.

Pfizer Laboratories. *Medical Economics.* November 1984.

Pines, Maya. "What You Eat Affects Your Brain." *Readers Digest.* September 1983, pp. 54-58.

Rapp, Doris J. *Is This Your Child?* New York: William Morrow and Co., Inc., 1991.

Restak, Richard. *The Brain.* New York: Bantam Books, 1984.

Ricketts, Max with Bien, Edwin. *The Great Anxiety Escape.* La Mesa, CA: Matulungin Publishing, 1990.

Rogers, Sherry A. *Tired or Toxic?* *Syracuse: Prestige Publishing,* 1990.

Sandler, M., et al. "Trace Amine Deficit In Depressive Illness: The Phenylalanine Connexion." *Acta Psychiatriaca Scandinavica Supplementation.* Vol. 280 1980, pp. 29-39.

Seyle, Hans. *Stress Without Distress.* New York: The New American Library, Inc. 1974, p. 36.

Slagle, Priscilla. *The Way Up From Down.* New York: St. Martin's Press, 1992.

Smith, Bernard H. and Rosich-Pla, Antonio. "The Biochemistry of Mental Illness." *Psychosomatics.* April 1979, pp. 278-283.

Smith, Lendon. *Feed Yourself Right.* New York: Dell Publishing Co., 1983.

"Tracking the Chemistry of Stress." *Time.* June 6, 1983, p. 51.

Van Baak, Alice. "Tryptophan-Natural Alternative to Tranquilizers." *Bestways.* October 1981, pp. 63-64.

Van Pelt, J.S., Ambrose, G. and Newbold G. *Medical Hypnosis Handbook.* Los Angeles: Wilshire Book Co., 1970.

Vnuk, John. "D-Phenylalanine the Pain Killer." *Health Express.* September 1983, p. 20.

------. "Phenylalanine." *Health Express.* July 1983, p. 26.

Watson, Robert L. *Current Concepts in Anesthesiology.* Symposia held at Brigham and Women's Hospital, Boston, MA, February 17, 1982.

Willliams, Roger J. and Kalita, Dwight K., eds. *A Physician's Handbook on Orthomolecular Medicine.* New Canaan, CN: Keats Publishing, Inc., 1977.

Zucker, Martin. " Orthomolecular Psychiatry Update." *Let's Live Magazine.* November, 1982, pp. 31-31.

Index

Call 1-800-669-CALM
--------------**To Order** --------------

Please Print

Name _____

Address _____

City _____ State _____ Zip _____

I would like to purchase	Price	Quantity	Total
Chronic Emotional Fatigue book	$3.95	_____	_____
The Anxiety Epidemic book (Dr. B.J. Sahley)	$9.95	_____	_____
Breaking Your Addiction Habit book (Drs. B.J. Sahley and K.Birkner)	$8.95	_____	_____
The Natural Way To Control Hyperactivity With Amino Acids and Nutrients (Dr. B.J. Sahley)	$6.95	_____	_____
Breaking the Sugar Addiction Cookbook (Kathy Birkner, C.R.N.A, Ph.D.)	$5.95	_____	_____
Anxiety Audio Cassette Tape (Dr. B.J. Sahley)	$10	_____	_____
Fear Audio Cassette Tape (Dr. B.J. Sahley)	$10	_____	_____
Phobias Audio Cassette Tape (Dr. B.J. Sahley)	$10	_____	_____
Anxiety / Panic Attacks Causes & Control Audio Cassette Tape (Dr. B.J. Sahley)	$10	_____	_____
Hyperactivity Causes & Control Audio Cassette Tape (Dr. B.J. Sahley)	$10	_____	_____
Communication Audio Cassette Tape (Dr. B.J. Sahley)	$10	_____	_____
Letting Go Audio Cassette Tape (Dr. B.J. Sahley)	$10	_____	_____
Guilt Audio Cassette Tape (Dr. B.J. Sahley)	$10	_____	_____
Being, Your Way Audio Cassette Tape (Dr. B. Sahley)	$10	_____	_____
Depression Audio Cassette Tape (Dr. B.J. Sahley)	$10	_____	_____
Anger Audio Cassette Tape (Dr. B.J. Sahley)	$10	_____	_____
Forgiving and Healing Audio Cassette (Dr. Sahley)	$10	_____	_____
Escape Audio Cassette Tape (Dr. B.J. Sahley)	$10	_____	_____
Orthomolecular Directory of Physicians and Therapists	$7.95	_____	_____
Catalog (No shipping charge)	$2	_____	_____
SUBTOTAL			_____
Texas Residents Add 8.25% Sales Tax			_____
**SHIPPING $3 first item and $1 subsequent			_____
TOTAL			_____

Personal checks are held for 10 days. To expediate order, send money order.

MC /Visa / Discover _ _ _ _ - _ _ _ _ - _ _ _ _ - _ _ _ _

Signature _____ Exp Date ___ / ___

Send To: **Pain & Stress Therapy Center**
5282 Medical Drive, Suite 160, San Antonio, TX 78229-6043

**Canadian & Other Foreign Countries ADD $5 to the above amounts. We accept U. S. World Money Orders or MC / Visa / Discover ONLY!

"Undefeated only because we have gone on trying."

T. S. Eliot

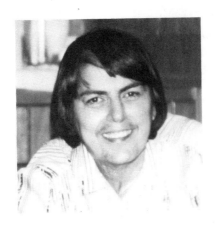

Billie J. Sahley, Ph.D. is Founder and Executive Director of the Pain & Stress Therapy Center in San Antonio, Texas. She is a Board Certified Medical Psychotherapist and Orthomolecular Therapist. She is a Diplomate in American Academy of Pain Management. Dr. Sahley is a graduate of the University of Texas, Clayton University School of Behavioral Medicine, and U.C.L.A. School of Integral Medicine. Additionally, she has studied advanced nutritional biochemistry through Jeffrey Bland, Ph.D. and HealthComm. She is a member of the Huxley Foundation, American Board of Medical Psychotherapists, Academy of Psychosomatic Medicine, American Academy of Pain Management, Sports Medicine Foundation, Academy of Environmental Medicine, American Association of Hypnotherapist, and American Mental Health Counselors Association. Dr. Sahley is also on the Scientific and Medical Advisory Board for Inter-Cal Corporation. She is author of *The Natural Way To Control Hyperactivity with Amino Acids and Nutrients* and *Chronic Emotional Fatigue,* co-author of *Breaking Your Addiction Habit,* and numerous audio cassette tapes. Dr. Sahley received a U.S. patent for both Calms Kids and SAF.

An example of the situational anxiety that may develop from childhood to adulthood is the case of the offspring of an alcoholic such as Paul in Chapter II. Paul was exposed day in and day out to his father's illness and experienced loss of control, anxiety, fear, and a constant feeling of uncertainty. As a child and then as an adult, he suffered from a continuous anxious state. Imagine the condition of the chemoreceptors in his brain; is it not possible that the day-in day-out fearful state could damage or make the chemoreceptors oversensitive and so misfire? This—or traumatic occurrences of various kinds—would create panic from fear whenever flashbacks of his childhood occurred, especially if one or both parents were physically abusive.

Considering that alcoholics are malnourished, the condition of their children would probably not be average. Since every cell in our body changes completely every six months, it is what we are able to absorb that determines our state of health. If the alcoholic does not receive or is unable to absorb the necessary nutrients, essential amino acids, and minerals, he/she—and his/her child will stay in a minus state of nutrition predisposing them to both physical and emotional illnesses.

The tranquilizers which are so often given to alcoholics' children to help them cope and sleep are nothing more than a sugar coating or possibly the beginning of their own addiction. The tranquilizers simply cover up the symptoms, but do not remove the cause.

In *Brain Allergies—The Psychonutrient Connection*, by William H. Philpott, M.D., and Dwight Kalita, Ph.D., the authors state that toximolecular psychiatrists (those who use drugs or synthetic substances not normally found in the human body) may think they are practicing scientific medicine, but they are not. Even though tranquilizers manage to control psychiatric symptoms, the underlying disease process initially responsible for the symptom usually remains unchecked.

Linus Pauling in defining "orthomolecular medicine" said that the treatment of disease is a matter of "varying the concentration of substances (i.e., the right molecules:

vitamins, minerals, trace elements, hormones, amino acids, enzymes) normally present in the human body." Through regulation of the concentration of chemical molecules, orthomolecular medicine aims at the achievement and preservation of optimum health and the prevention and treatment of disease.

Many physicians are unfamiliar with the orthomolecular approach and know only the drug or toximolecular approach. Dr. Philpott states that "drugs are chemical substances which, even if given singly, radically alter man's metabolic machinery and many times interfere with normal vitamin, mineral, amino-acids and enzyme activities in the body. Nutrients, on the other hand, working as a team, act constructively as building blocks for life in general; without them, human life could not exist. Life can exist without drugs!"

Abram Hoffer, M.D., Ph.D., an orthomolecular psychiatrist, has warned that he has seen many hyperactive young children that were placed on symptomatic drug therapy such as Ritalin. This type of therapy brings hyperactive symptoms emotionally under control, but later the patient degenerates further into adult schizophrenia; the adult schizophrenia results because the underlying metabolic cause remains untreated.

Toximolecular medicine requires only one thing from its patients—that they continue to take their drugs or tranquilizers. It is disturbing to think that these patients on drugs often have to pay an extremely high price for their symptomatic relief; they run the statistically high risk of becoming permanently incarcerated and/or controlled by their chemical straitjackets.

Hoffer and Walker in *Orthomolecular Nutrition* offer the following summary:

> Every tissue of the body is affected by nutrition. Under conditions of poor nutrition the kidney stops filtering, the stomach stops digesting, the adrenals stop secreting, and other organs follow suit. Unfortunately, some psychiatrists labor under the false belief that somehow brain func-

tion is completely unaffected by nutrition. It seems that many psychiatrists and their parapsychiatric colleagues such as psychologists and social workers consider the brain is not an organ of the body that needs nourishment.

I repeat once more—**there is no such thing as a tranquilizer deficiency.**

Symptoms of Anxiety

The following are some of the anxiety-fear-panic-phobia symptoms that have shown improvement with orthomolecular therapy:

1. Feeling a loss of control
2. Going insane
3. Light-headedness, faint
4. Unsteady legs
5. Difficulty in breathing—unable to take a deep breath
6. Fear of heart attack
7. Heart pounding, skipping, racing
8. Constant fear of dying
9. Tingling lips and fingers
10. Stomach pain, diarrhea, constipation, nausea, bottomlessness
11. Excessive sweating, hot or cold
12. Headaches, neck and shoulder pain
13. Low back pain
14. Tender-headedness
15. Feeling tired, weak, no energy
16. Feeling as though you are outside your body
17. Mood and emotion swings
18. Unable to sleep
19. Restless sleep; nightmares
20. Unable to relax
21. Anxiety, tension, restless
22. Depressing or negative thought pattern
23. Need to have someone around constantly
24. Rush of panic or fear for no reason

25. Fear of crowds, can't breathe
26. Emotional eating, food won't go down
27. Muscle twitching
28. Unable to remember
29. Withdrawal to home
30. Dry cotton mouth
31. Blurred vision
32. Mental confusion

Formula for Natural Diet Supplement

According to Roger J. Williams in *Nutrition Against Disease*, "an alcoholic should supplement his diet with a good assortment of minerals and vitamins—even amino acids," since his years of drinking have typically caused malnourishment. A natural nutritional formula consists of a number of vitamins, minerals, amino acids, and herbs to assist the alcoholic in his nutritional recovery. The formula of this typical therapeutic replacement for toxic prescription drugs consists of the following substances.

AMINO ACIDS

These are the building blocks for our *proteins*. Proteins are essential for a number of reasons:

1. They furnish amino acids required for building of body tissues and health.
2. They supply food fuel for the body whenever insufficient fats and carbohydrates are consumed; they also help to maintain normal blood sugar.
3. They assist in the transport of various minerals and vitamins.
4. They assist in the acid-base balance of the body.

Protein is needed for the health and formation of muscles, hormones, membranes, glands, enzymes, skin, plasma, teeth, antibodies, ligaments, hair, fingernails, bones, cartilage, hemoglobin, brain cells, and nerve cells.

Signs and symptoms of insufficient protein intake include: fatigue, poor digestion, bloating, slow growth, anemia, low vitality, sluggish pulse, scarring and slow heal-